Handbook of Pharmacology for
THE ANESTHESIOLOGISTS

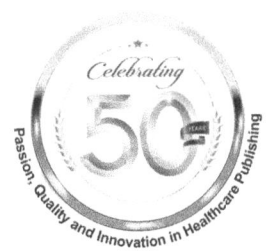

Handbook of Pharmacology for
THE ANESTHESIOLOGISTS

Lopamudra Chowdhury
MBBS DA MD (Pharmacology)
Associate Professor and Head
Department of Pharmacology
Murshidabad Medical College
Murshidabad, West Bengal, India

Foreword
Manjushree Ray

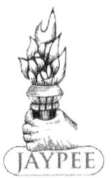

JAYPEE BROTHERS MEDICAL PUBLISHERS
The Health Sciences Publisher
New Delhi | London | Panama

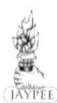 **Jaypee Brothers Medical Publishers (P) Ltd.**

Headquarters
Jaypee Brothers Medical Publishers (P) Ltd
4838/24, Ansari Road, Daryaganj
New Delhi 110 002, India
Phone: +91-11-43574357
Fax: +91-11-43574314
Email: jaypee@jaypeebrothers.com

Overseas Offices

J.P. Medical Ltd
83 Victoria Street, London
SW1H 0HW (UK)
Phone: +44 20 3170 8910
Fax: +44 (0)20 3008 6180
Email: info@jpmedpub.com

Jaypee-Highlights Medical Publishers Inc
City of Knowledge, Bld. 235, 2nd Floor
Clayton, Panama City, Panama
Phone: +1 507-301-0496
Fax: +1 507-301-0499
Email: cservice@jphmedical.com

Jaypee Brothers Medical Publishers (P) Ltd
Bhotahity, Kathmandu, Nepal
Phone: +977-9741283608
Email: kathmandu@jaypeebrothers.com

Website: www.jaypeebrothers.com
Website: www.jaypeedigital.com

© 2019, Jaypee Brothers Medical Publishers

The views and opinions expressed in this book are solely those of the original contributor(s)/author(s) and do not necessarily represent those of editor(s) of the book.

All rights reserved. No part of this publication may be reproduced, stored or transmitted in any form or by any means, electronic, mechanical, photocopying, recording or otherwise, without the prior permission in writing of the publishers.

All brand names and product names used in this book are trade names, service marks, trademarks or registered trademarks of their respective owners. The publisher is not associated with any product or vendor mentioned in this book.

Medical knowledge and practice change constantly. This book is designed to provide accurate, authoritative information about the subject matter in question. However, readers are advised to check the most current information available on procedures included and check information from the manufacturer of each product to be administered, to verify the recommended dose, formula, method and duration of administration, adverse effects and contraindications. It is the responsibility of the practitioner to take all appropriate safety precautions. Neither the publisher nor the author(s)/editor(s) assume any liability for any injury and/or damage to persons or property arising from or related to use of material in this book.

This book is sold on the understanding that the publisher is not engaged in providing professional medical services. If such advice or services are required, the services of a competent medical professional should be sought.

Every effort has been made where necessary to contact holders of copyright to obtain permission to reproduce copyright material. If any have been inadvertently overlooked, the publisher will be pleased to make the necessary arrangements at the first opportunity. The **CD/DVD-ROM** (if any) provided in the sealed envelope with this book is complimentary and free of cost. **Not meant for sale.**

Inquiries for bulk sales may be solicited at: jaypee@jaypeebrothers.com

Handbook of Pharmacology for the Anesthesiologists

First Edition: **2019**

ISBN: 978-93-5270-679-2

Dedicated to

All my respected teachers till date, my friends and associates of Anesthesiology

My husband Tamonas and my beloved son Anurag

Foreword

Pharmacology has been an integral part of Anesthesiology from its inception. Pharmacological agents are exclusively used in day-to-day anesthesiology practice. Drugs consumed by patients for coexisting diseases often have significant interactions with different anesthetic agents. Knowledge of the basic mechanisms, pharmacokinetics, pharmacodynamics and their alterations in various scenarios is essential to develop a solid foundation in the practices of anesthesiology.

Most of the textbooks of anesthesiology have failed to address pharmacology in detail from the anesthesiologist point of view, especially from an Indian perspective. In this book, this dearth has been satisfied by a renowned pharmacologist, who also has a vast knowledge in the field of anesthesiology. Dr Lopamudra Chowdhury, a renowned teacher of pharmacology with an immense experience in the field of anesthesia has developed a solid foundation in this book on which the learners can integrate their knowledge.

Handbook of Pharmacology for the Anesthesiologists covers the entire subject relevant to anesthesia practice in 21 chapters. Chapter one is primarily designed to discuss basic pharmacology and, chapters 2 to 10 have covered anesthesia related drugs. Chapters 11 to 19 have included various pharmacological agents either used by anesthesiologist to prevent or treat complications or used by patients for their some pre-existing illness. Chapters 20 and 21 are discussions about some special and emergency scenarios.

All efforts have been made by the author in providing accurate and up-to-date information. *Handbook of Pharmacology for the Anesthesiologists* is a complete package of pharmacology for students, teachers and the specialists of anesthesiology.

Manjushree Ray
MBBS MD MAMS MBA
Principal and Professor
Department of Anesthesiology
Calcutta Medical College
Kolkata, West Bengal, India

Preface

The practice of anesthesia is intricately dependent on the use of drugs. The knowledge of pharmacology regarding anesthetic drugs as well as other systemic drugs is essential for proper administration of anesthesia and avoidence of catastrophe. As Anesthesiologists are ever busy, this book is intended to be concise yet highly informative and user friendly. This book additionally provides quick information of drug doses, adverse effects, contraindications of use and special precautions which has to be undertaken during therapy. The contents will be especially helpful not only for the students, but also for the busy practitioners. The clinical pearls and the comparative study of drugs discussed at the end of the chapters are for instant overview. Some chapters as in 'Drugs of the Cardiovascular System' or 'Drug Therapy in Special Cases', have been duly stressed and would be of immense help. Though the book has been named, *The Handbook of Pharmacology for the Anesthesiologists*, this book precisely covers almost all important chapters of Pharmacology and would provide important at hand information for postgraduate aspirants too for their entrance examinations.

I hope, this book will save time yet provide important information. I would highly appreciate any feedback regarding this endeavor.

Lopamudra Chowdhury

Acknowledgments

First and foremost I would like to acknowledge the guidance and advice of my teacher, Prof Anupam Goswami, who had given his valuable time to go through each and every chapter of this book. I would also acknowledge Prof Manjushree Ray, who in spite of her extremely busy schedule had given her valuable time to go through the chapters. I am thankful to Prof Indranil Biswas, Prof Dipasri Bhattacharya, Dr Anjana and Dr Debanjali for their valuable opinions regarding this book. Last but not least, I would like to thank my family members for their constant support without whom this effort would not have been successful. I am also indebted to Mr Sabyasachi and team Jaypee Brothers Medical Publishers, New Delhi, India, for their help.

Contents

1. **General Pharmacology** — 1
   - Some Terminologies *1* • Bioavailability *2*
   - Drug Antagonism *6* • Drug Agonism *8*
   - Muscarinic Cholinergic Receptors *9* • Ion Channel Receptors *13*
   - Biotransformation *15* • Second Messengers *18*
   - Adverse Drug Reactions *19*

2. **General Anesthetics** — 24
   - History *24* • Physiological Effects of General Anesthetics *24*
   - Components of General Anesthesia *25*
   - Minimum Alveolar Concentration *25*
   - Mechanism of Anesthesia *27*
   - General Principles of Inhalational Anesthesia *27*
   - Clinical Signs of Anesthesia (Based on Ether Anesthesia) *27*

   Common Anesthetics — 29
   - Halothane *29* • Isoflurane *30* • Enflurane *31*
   - Desflurane *31* • Sevoflurane *32* • Nitrous Oxide *32*
   - Xenon *33* • Therapeutic Gases *34*

3. **Parenteral Anesthetics** — 35
   - Ideal Anesthetic (IV) agent *35* • Barbiturates *36*
   - Propofol *37* • Etomidate *38* • Ketamine *39*
   - Midazolam *41* • Fentanyl *41*
   - Total Intravenous Anesthesia *42* • Conscious Sedation *44*
   - Role of α_2-Receptor Agonists (Clonidine and Dexmedetomidine) in Anesthesia *44*

4. **Hypnotics and Sedatives** — 46
   - Definitions *46* • History *46* • Classification *46*
   - Mechanism of Action *47* • Benzodiazepines *47*
   - Barbiturates *49* • Newer Hypnotics *50* • Buspirone *51*
   - Comparative Study of Commonly Used Drugs *51*

5. **Skeletal Muscle Relaxants** — 53
   - Classification *53*
   - Features Common to All Muscle Relaxants *53*
   - Pharmacokinetics *54*

6. **Drugs Used in Reversal of Neuromuscular Block** — 61
   - History *61* • Classification *61* • Mechanism of Action *61*
   - Pharmacokinetics *62*

7. **Anticholinergic Drugs Used in Anesthesia** — 65
   - Actions of Prototype Drug Atropine *65*
   - Pharmacokinetics *66* • Preanesthetic Medications *67*

8. Nonsteroidal Anti-inflammatory Drugs — 68
- History *68* • Pathophysiology *68*
- Classification *69* • Mechanism of Action *69* • Aspirin *70*
- Other Salicylates in Use *72*
- Acetaminophen (Paracetamol) *72*
- Indomethacin *73* • Sulindac *73* • Tolmetin *74*
- Ketorolac *74* • Nabumetone *74* • Diclofenac *74*
- Ibuprofen *74* • Other Propionic Acid Derivatives *75*
- COX-2 Selective NSAIDs *75*
- Comparative Study of Some Commonly Used Analgesics *76*
- Patient-controlled Analgesia *77*
- Common Adverse Effects of NSAIDs *77*

9. Centrally Acting Analgesics/Opioids — 78
- Endogenous Opioid System *78* • Opioid Receptors *79*
- Codeine *82* • Pethidine/Meperidine *82* • Fentanyl *83*
- Remifentanil *83* • Methadone *83* • Tramadol *83*
- Uses of Morphine and Congeners *84* • Agonist Antagonists *84*
- Opioid Antagonists *85* • Drug Interaction *86*
- Points to Note *86*

10. Local Anesthetics — 87
- History *87* • Structure *87*
- Mechanism of Action *88* • Pharmacokinetics *88*
- Cocaine *89* • Lidocaine *89* • Bupivacaine *89*
- Clinical Preparation *90* • Features of Amide LA *91*
- Molecular Mechanism of Action *94* • Regional Anesthesia *94*
- Epidural Block *99*

11. Drugs Used in Nausea and Vomiting — 101
- Classification *101*
- Comparative Study of Commonly Used Drugs *108*

12. Drugs Used in Peptic Ulcer Disease — 109
- Classification *109* • H_2 Antagonists *110*
- Proton Pump Inhibitors *111* • Prostaglandin Analogs *112*
- Sucralfate *113* • Colloidal Bismuth *113* • Antacids *114*

13. Drugs Used in Treatment of Asthma — 115
Drugs for Bronchial Asthma — 115
- Definition *115*
- Classification of Drugs Used in Bronchial Asthma *116*
- Sympathomimetics *118* • Methylxanthines *120*
- Anticholinergics *122* • Glucocorticoids *122*
- Mast Cell Stabilizers *123*
- Leukotriene Pathway Inhibitors *123*
- K^+ Channel Openers *124*
- Treatment of Status Asthmaticus/Acute Severe Asthma *125*

14. Drugs Used in Cough — 126
- Pharyngeal Demulcents *127*
- Expectorants/Mucokinetics *127* • Mucolytics *127*
- Antitussives *127*

15. Drugs Acting in Cardiovascular System — 129

Pathophysiology of Shock and its Management — 129
- Types of Shock *129* • Compensatory Mechanisms *130*
- Treatment *130*

Vasodilators — 134
- Sodium Nitroprusside *134* • Glyceryl Trinitrate *135*
- Hydralazine *136* • Minoxidil *137*
- Vasodilators in Heart Failure *137*

β-Blockers — 140
- Classification *140* • Pharmacokinetics *141*
- Pharmacodynamics *142* • Uses of β-Blockers *143*
- Adverse Effects *143* • β-Blockers in Heart Failure *144*

Inotropic Agents and Vasoconstrictors — 146
- Adrenaline *146* • Noradrenaline *147* • Dopamine *147*
- Dobutamine *148* • Phenylephrine *148*
- Mephentermine *149* • Metaraminol *149*
- Midodrine *149* • Milrinone *149*

Drugs used in Hypertension — 151
- Causes *151* • Treatment *152* • Indications for Therapy *153*
- Blood Pressure Management Protocol *153*

Drugs Used in Ischemic Heart Disease — 160
- Drugs Used in Angina *160*
- Drug Therapy in Acute Myocardial Infarction *160*
- Clinical Pearl *161*

Diuretics — 162
- Osmotic Diuretics *164*
- Vasopressin Antagonists *165*

Pathophysiology of Renin–Angiotensin System — 166
- Components of Renin-Angiotensin System *166*

ACE Inhibitors — 170
- Characteristics *170* • Adverse Effects *171*

Angiotensin II Receptor Blockers (ARBs) — 172
- Actions *172* • Advantages *172* • Characteristics *172*

Calcium Channel Blockers — 173
- Mechanism of Action *173* • Verapamil *175*
- Cilnidipine *175*

Cardiac Glycosides — 176
- Mechanism of Action *176*

Cardiac Dysrhythmia and Antiarrhythmics — 178
- First-degree AV Heart Block *178*
- Second-degree AV Heart Block *178*
- Third-degree AV Heart Block *179*
- Wolff-Parkinson White Syndrome (Preexcitation Syndrome) *183*
- Lown–Ganong–Levine Syndrome *184*
- Classification of Antiarrhythmic Drugs *185*

16. Anticoagulants, Fibrinolytics and Antiplatelet Agents — 187
- Anticoagulants *187*
- Heparin Antagonist (Protamine Sulfate) *191*
- Platelet Inhibitors *191* • Fibrinolytics *193*

17. Drugs Used in Central Nervous System — 195
Drugs Used in Parkinsonism — 195
- Levodopa *195* • Dopamine Receptor Agonists *196*
- COMT Inhibitors *197* • Selective MAO Inhibitors *197*
- Muscarinic Receptor Antagonists *198*
- Drug-induced Parkinsonism *198*

Antidepressants — 200
- Mechanism of Action *201*
- Long-term Effects of Antidepressants *201*

Anesthetic Implications in Patients on Antiepileptic Drugs — 205

18. Drugs Acting on Endocrine System — 206
Antidiabetic Drugs — 206
- Preoperative Glycemic Goals *206*
- Insulin in Treatment of Diabetes *206*
- Methods of Insulin Therapy *207* • Diabetic Ketoacidosis *207*
- Hyperosmolar Nonketotic Coma *207*
- Hypoglycemia *208* • Oral Antidiabetic Agents *208*

Drugs Used In Thyroid Disorders — 211
- Antithyroid Drugs *211*

19. Oxygen Therapy and Humidification — 213
- Indications *213* • Techniques of Oxygen Therapy *213*
- Toxicity *215* • Humidification *215* • Antioxidants *217*

20. Drug Therapy in Special Cases — 218
The Pediatric Patients — 218
- Physiology in the Neonate and Pediatric Patients *218*
- Pharmacology of Anesthetic Drugs *221*

Patient with Chronic Renal Failure — 222
- Features Associated with Chronic Renal Failure *222*
- Preoperative Preparation *222* • Postoperative Follow-up *224*
- Dose Calculation in Impaired Renal Function *224*

Patient With Liver Dysfunction   225
- Pathophysiological Changes Associated with Chronic Liver Disease *225*
- Preoperative Preparation *225*
- Postoperative Follow-up *226*

The Elderly Patient   227
- Age-related Changes in Pharmacokinetics and Pharmacodynamics *227*
- Drugs with Reduced Renal or Hepatic Elimination in the Elderly *228*

21. Management of Emergency Situations   229
- Acute Severe Asthma *229*
- Hypertensive Crisis *229*
- Severe Laryngospasm *230*
- Pulmonary Edema *231*
- Malignant Hyperthermia *231*
- Raised Intracranial Pressure *231*
- Acute Adrenal Crisis *231*
- Thyroid Storm *232*
- Cardiac Arrest *232*

Bibliography   234

Index   *235*

CHAPTER 1

General Pharmacology

SOME TERMINOLOGIES

The term *pharmacon* means drugs; *logos* means studies.
Pharmacology is a branch of medicine which deals with drugs.

Drug (WHO)

Drug is a chemical substance or biological product that is used or intended to be used to modify or explore physiological systems or pathological states for the benefit of the recipient.

Drug is called medicine when used in proper dosage form for safe administration. All medicines are drugs but all drugs are not medicines.

Active Principle of Drug

Chemical constituent present in the drug which is responsible for pharmacological effect of the drug, e.g. alkaloids pilocarpine, atropine, physostigmine, quinine, etc.

Names of Drug

A drug may be named in various ways: chemical, generic or nonproprietory, proprietory, e.g. chemical name—acetaminophen or 4-acetamidophenol generic/nonproprietory name—Paracetamol, proprietory/trade name—Calpol.

Determination of Drug Routes

Routes of drug administration is determined primarily by—
- Properties of the drug, e.g. water or lipid solubility, degree of ionization, molecular weight, etc.
- Therapeutic objectives, e.g. rapidity of onset of action, duration, site of action, etc.
- Patient profile whether patient is conscious/unconscious, compliant/noncompliant, age of the patient, whether patient is vomiting/not vomiting (Flowchart 1.1 and Fig. 1.1).

Flowchart 1.1: Routes of drug administration.

Enteral	Parenteral	Others
1. Oral	1. Intravascular	1. Inhalation
2. Sublingual	– intravenous	2. Intranasal
3. Rectal	– intra-arterial	3. Intrathecal/ intraventricular
	2. Intramuscular	4. Topical
	3. Subcutaneous	5. Intra-articular
	4. Intradermal	
	5. Transdermal	

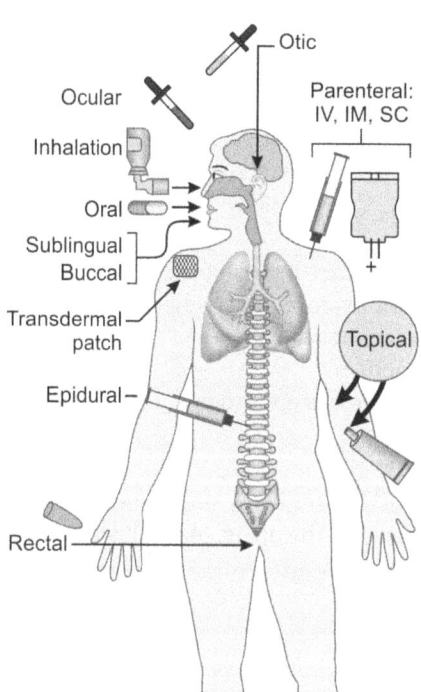

Figure 1.1: Various routes of drug application.

BIOAVAILABILITY

It is the measure of the fraction of administered dose of a drug that reaches the systemic circulation in the unchanged form. Bioavailability (BA) is related to the rate and extent of absorption of a drug from its dosage form. Bioavailability of IV (intravenous) administered drug is 100% but it is not so, when administered orally. By plotting plasma concentrations of the drug vs time, one can measure area under the curve. This curve reflects the extent of absorption of the drug (Figs. 1.2A and B). So, bioavailability of a drug administered orally is the ratio of area under the curve calculated for oral administration compared with the area under the curve calculated for intravenous (IV) injection (Fig. 1.3).

Bioavailability of an orally administered drug can be assessed by the following (expressed as %):

$$BA = \frac{\text{Area under the curve for oral administration}}{\text{area under the curve for IV administration}}$$

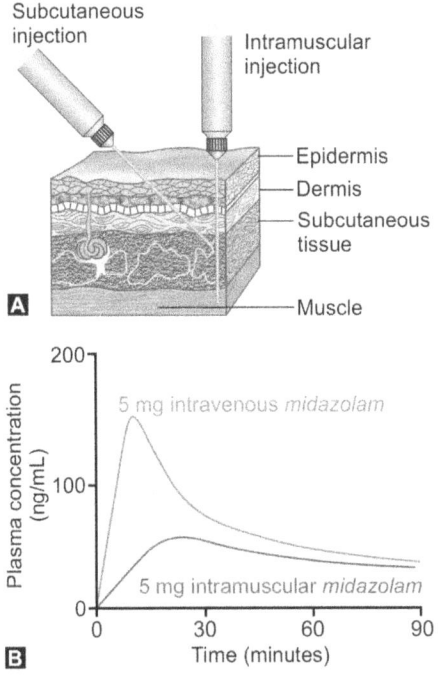

Figures 1.2A and B: Bioavailability of drug midazolam.

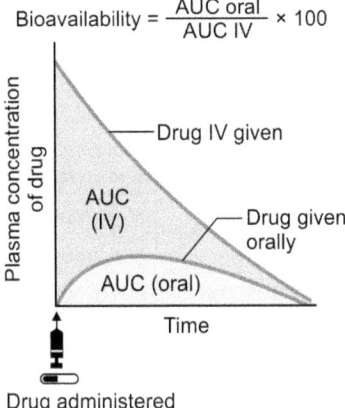

Figure 1.3: Diagram comparing BA of various routes.
AUC: area under the curve; IV: intravenous; BA: bioavailability

Significance

- Variation in bioavailability affects drugs with narrow safety margin, toxicity may be precipitated.
- It influences the therapeutic efficacy of drugs, specially antibiotics.
- Enteric coated tablets are used to increase bioavailability of drugs destroyed by enzymes in GIT. Hence, route of administration and dosage form to be decided accordingly.

Factors that Influence Bioavailability

- First-pass hepatic metabolism—Drug absorbed from GIT enters portal circulation, before entering systemic circulation. If it is partly metabolized by the hepatic enzymes the amount of unchanged drug reaching systemic circulation is decreased, e.g. propranolol, lidocaine have high first pass hepatic metabolism.
- Solubility of drug—Hydrophilic drugs are poorly absorbed. Again extremely hydrophobic substitutes too are not absorbed because they are insoluble in aqueous body fluids.
- Chemical stability—Some drugs are destroyed in the GIT by degradative enzymes.
- pH of the drug—Some drugs are unstable at gastric pH.
- Properties of the drug and dosage form—Particle size, salt form, crystal polymorphism and presence of excipients (binders and dispersing agents) can influence rate of dissolution.
- Presence of food or other drugs—These influence the absorption of the drug.
- GI motility—It affects drug absorption hence bioavailability.

Two related drugs are bioequivalent if they show comparable bioavailability and similar times to achieve peak blood concentration. Two similar drugs which are bioequivalent may not be therapeutically equivalent.

Safety Profile of a Drug

A drug can be termed "risk free" if the precise action of the drug is known by the physician; drug was used correctly in appropriate dose and for

Route	Bioavailability (%)	Characteristics
Intravenous (IV)	100	Most rapid onset
Intramuscular (IM)	75 ≤ 100	Injection may be painful
Subcutaneous (SC)	75 ≤ 100	Injection may be painful
Oral	5 <100	Significant first-pass metabolism
Rectal	30 to <100	Less first-pass metabolism than oral
Inhalation	5 to <100	Rapid onset
Transdermal	80 to <100	Slow onset

appropriate indication; drug had biological selectivity or administered by selective targeted delivery.

The criteria of a risk-free drug is never achieved because—
- Drugs are not usually selective.
- If the action is selective, its action may be extended to other sites.
- Prolonged administration of a drug can lead to functional (receptor modification) and organic (iatrogenic disease) changes.
- Genetic variability may induce unpredictable responses.
- Need for dosage monitoring and adjustment.
- Physiological variables like age, sex, pregnancy, lactation affect disposition of a drug.
- Pathological variability, e.g. renal or hepatic disease also influences drug level.
- Ignorant and casual prescribing may be responsible for iatrogenic disease conditions.

Methods to Ensure Safety of Drug
- Target-oriented drug delivery.
- Therapeutic dose monitoring.
- Pharmacovigilance of adverse drug reactions (ADR).
- Proper information to the patient regarding the usage details.
- It is advisable not to prescribe a drug about which the prescriber is not fully conversant.

First-pass Metabolism

Most of the drugs administered orally, after absorption from the gastro-intestinal tract (GIT), enters the portal circulation first before reaching the systemic circulation. As the drug gains access to the liver via the portal circulation, it is exposed to the drug metabolizing enzymes (also in the intestinal wall) of the liver and a considerable fraction of the administered dose is metabolized. This metabolism is called first-pass metabolism.

Sites of First-pass Metabolism
(a) Intestine, (b) liver (mainly), (c) skin, (d) lungs.

The extent of first-pass metabolism differs for different drugs and is an important determinant of oral bioavailability. Consequences of first-pass metabolism—
1. Oral dose required is higher than sublingual or parenteral route.
2. There is marked individual variation in bioavailability, depending on the extent of metabolism.
3. Oral bioavailability is increased in severe liver disease.
4. Oral bioavailability is increased if another drug competing with it in first-pass metabolism is administered concurrently, e.g. chlorpromazine and propranolol.

Examples

Examples of drugs with high first-pass metabolism—isoprenaline, lignocaine, hydrocortisone, testosterone, propranolol, nitroglycerin and verapamil, etc.

Hence, these drugs with high first pass metabolism should either be given in high oral dose or preferably oral administration should be avoided. Routes which bypass first-pass metabolism are preferred.

Routes which Bypass First-pass Metabolism

- Parenteral → IV, IM, SC and routes like intravenous intramuscular, or subcutaneous.
- Sublingual.
- Transdermal.
- Topical.

DRUG ANTAGONISM

When one drug decreases or inhibits the action of the other, they are said to be antagonists. The types of antagonism may be classified according to mechanism as—(a) chemical antagonism, (b) pharmacokinetic antagonism, (c) antagonism by receptor block and (d) physiological antagonism—e.g. insulin and glucose on blood glucose level.

Chemical Antagonism

Condition where two substances combine in solution, as a result of which the effect of active drug is lost, e.g. thiopentone + succinylcholine → precipitate. Drug chemical interaction leads to drug inactivation formation.

Pharmacokinetic Antagonism

In this antagonism, antagonist effectively reduces the concentration of active drug at the site of action, either by affecting drug absorption, increasing the rate of metabolism or increasing the rate of renal excretion of the active drug.

Antagonism by Receptor Block

It is of two types; competitive and noncompetitive. In competitive receptor antagonism. Drug reception is blocked by antagonist either reversibly or irreversibly (Flowchart 1.2 and Fig. 1.4).

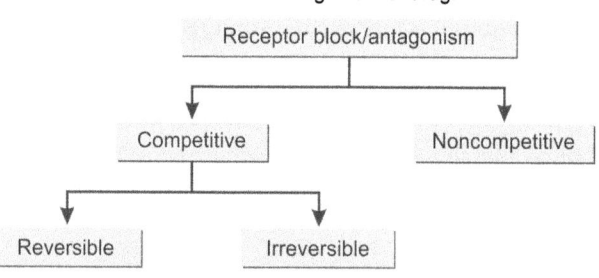

Flowchart 1.2: Antagonism of drug.

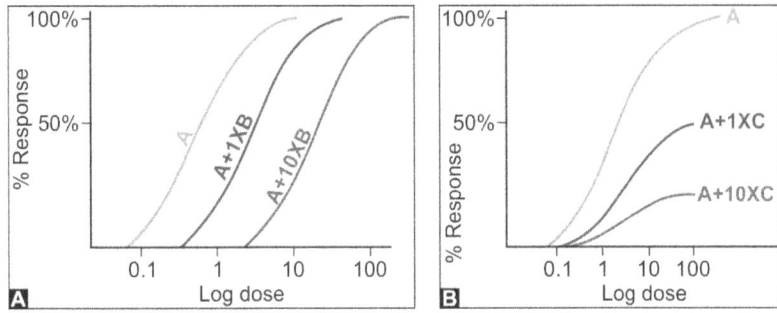

Figures 1.4A and B: Diagram of drug antagonism. (A) Competitive; (B) Noncompetitive.

Competitive Antagonism
- Antagonist binds with the same receptor as the agonist.
- Antagonist resembles chemically with the agonist.
- Intensity of response depends on the concentration of both agonist and antagonist.

Reversible antagonism: The antagonist has affinity for the same receptor as the agonist but lacks efficacy.
- Parallel shift of the agonist log dose concentration-effect curve without any decrease in the maximal response.
- Rate of dissociation of the antagonist molecule is sufficiently high.
- New equilibrium is rapidly established on addition of the agonist.

Irreversible antagonism: The antagonist bears high affinity to the receptor and binds with strong covalent bonds so that it cannot be detached easily.
- Antagonism is not surmountable.
- Antagonist dissociates very slowly.
- No change in antagonist occupancy takes place when agonist is applied.
- Reactive grouping of drug binds covalently to receptor.

Noncompetitive Antagonism
- Chemical structure of the antagonist is not similar to that of the agonist and binds to an allosteric site.
- Binds to another site of receptor.
- Does not resemble the agonist.
- Flattening of agonist drug response curve (DRC).
- Maximum response is suppressed.
- Response depends on concentration of antagonist.

Physiological/Functional Antagonism
The two drugs act on different receptors or by different mechanisms but have opposite effects on the same physiological function, e.g. glucagon and insulin on blood sugar level, ACE inhibitor and thiazide diuretic on serum potassium level.

Flowchart 1.3: Types of drug agonism.

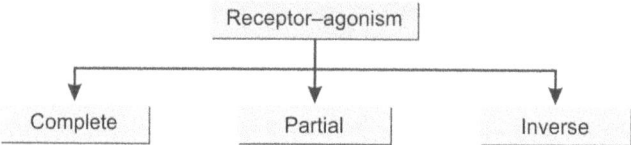

DRUG AGONISM (FLOWCHART 1.3)

- *Full agonists*: Agonists which can produce maximum effects and have high efficacy.
- *Partial agonists*: Agonists which produce submaximal effects and have intermediate efficacy.
- *Inverse agonists*: It shows selectivity for the receptor but produces effect opposite to that of an agonist. Hence shows affinity but negative efficacy.

Agonists on binding to receptors initiate changes in cell function, to bring about various effects. Potency of an agonist depends on two parameters—
- *Affinity*: Ability to bind to receptors.
- *Efficacy*: Ability to initiate changes that bring about effects.

According to the two state model, agonists show selectivity for the activated state of the receptor while antagonists show no selectivity.

Drugs act on various types of receptors:
- G-protein coupled receptor (GPCR)—e.g. adrenergic, muscarinic receptors (cholinergic).
- Ion-channel receptor—e.g. nicotinic (cholinergic), $GABA_A$, $5HT_3$, receptors.
- Transmembrane enzyme linked receptor—e.g. insulin, epidermal growth factor, nerve growth factor receptor.
- Transmembrane JAK-STAT binding receptor e.g. growth hormone, prolactin receptor.
- Nuclear receptor—e.g. steroids hormones, vitamin D.

G-protein Coupled Receptor

The G-protein coupled receptors are also known as metabotropic receptors or seven transmembrane spanning (heptahelical) receptors. They are membrane receptors that are coupled to intracellular effector system via G-protein. They constitute the largest family and include receptors for many hormones and slow transmitters.

G-protein coupled receptor (GPCR) consists of a single polypeptide chain of up to 1100 residues; the characteristic structure comprises seven transmembrane α-helices, with extracellular N-terminal domain of varying length and an intracellular C-terminal domain.

G-protein coupled receptor (GPCR) are divided into 3 distinct families. They share the same heptahelical structure but differ in other respects, e.g. length of the N-terminus—location of the agonist binding domain.

- *Family A*: Related to rhodopsin, most monoamine and neuropeptide receptors. It is by far the largest.
- *Family C*: The smallest, its main members being the metabotropic glutamate receptors and the Ca^{+2} sensitizing receptors.
- *Family B*: Secretin/glucagon receptor family. Receptors for peptide hormones including secretin, glucagon, calcitonin.

Examples: Muscarinic cholinergic receptors, adrenoceptors, chemokine receptors, neuropeptide receptors. The first G-protein coupled receptor (GPCR) to be fully characterized was the β-adrenoceptor which was cloned in 1986. So far, G-protein coupled receptor (GPCR) cannot be obtained in crystalline form, so powerful techniques of X-ray crystallography cannot yet be used to define the molecular structure of the receptors in detail.

The long third cytoplasmic loop is the region of the molecule that couples to the G-protein. Usually a particular receptor subtype couples selectively with a particular G-protein, swapping parts of the cytoplasmic loop between different receptors alters their G-protein selectivity. For small molecules such as nor adrenaline the ligand binding domain appears to reside not on the extracellular N-terminal region but buried in the cleft between the α-helical segments within the membrane. Peptide ligands such as substance P, bind more superficially to the extracellular loops.

Though activation of G-protein coupled receptor (GPCR) is normally the consequence of agonist binding, it can occur by other mechanism.
- Rhodopsin activated by light induced cis-trans isomerization.
- Thrombin initiates a variety of cellular response by binding to a GPCR.
- β-adrenoceptor—mutations in the third intracellular loop or simply overexpression of the receptor, result in constitutive receptor activation.

Inactivation occurs by desensitization involving phosphorylation after which the receptor is internalized and degraded to be replaced by newly synthesized protein. One of the intracellular loops is larger than the others and interacts with the G-protein. The G-protein is a membrane protein compromising three subunits (α, β, γ), the α subunit possessing guanosine triphosphate (GTP) ase activity. The α subunits of G-proteins differ in structure.

Coupling of the α-subunit to an agonist occupied receptor causes the bound guanosine diphosphate (GDP) to exchange with intracellular guanosine triphosphate (GTP), The α-GTP complex then dissociates from the receptor and from the βγ subunit complex and interacts with a target protein (target 1). The βγ complex may also activate a target protein (target 2). Guanosine triphosphate (GTP) ase activity of the α–subunit is increased when the target protein is bound, leading to hydrolysis of the bound guanosine triphosphate (GTP) to guanosine diphosphate (GDP), where upon the α-subunit reunites with the βγ complex.

MUSCARINIC CHOLINERGIC RECEPTORS

Two classes of receptors for acetylcholine are recognized—muscarinic and nicotinic. The muscarinic receptors are G-protein coupled receptor (GPCR) and are selectively stimulated by muscarine and blocked by atropine (Fig. 1.5).

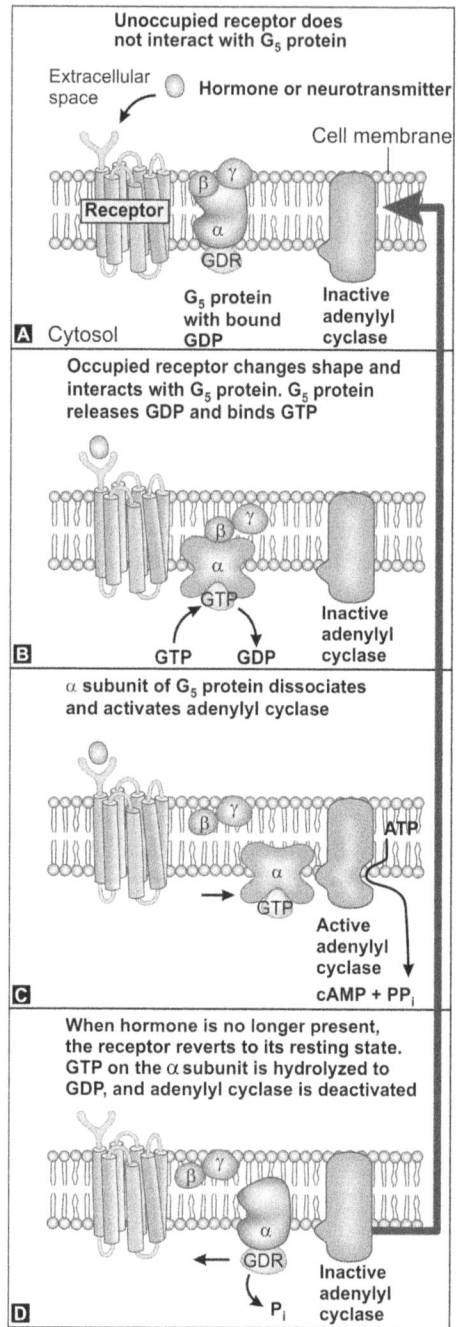

Figures 1.5A to D: Diagram of G-protein coupled receptor (GPCR).
GDP: guanosine diphosphate; GTP: guanosine triphosphate; cAMP: cyclic adenosine monophosphate

- *Sites*: These receptors are primarily present on autonomic effector cells in periphery—heart, blood vessels, eye, smooth muscles, glands of GI, respiratory and urinary tract and sweat glands.
- *CNS*: Preganglionic nerve fibers, ganglia—modulatory role.
- *History*: Muscarinic receptors were characterized initially by analysis of the responses of cells and tissues in the periphery and the CNS. Differential effects of two muscarinic antagonists, bethanechol and MeN-A 343 on the tone of esophageal sphincter led to the initial designation M_1 and M_2 (effector cell) by Goyal and Rattan 1978. Subsequently, radiological binding studies definitively revealed distinct populations of antagonist binding sites.
- *Types*: By pharmacological as well as molecular cloning techniques, muscarinic receptors have been divided into 5 subtypes—M_1, M_2, M_3, M_4 and M_5. The first 3 subtypes have been functionally characterized but responses mediated by M_4 and M_5 subtypes are not well defined.

M_1 Receptors

- **Main locations—CNS**: cortex, hippocampus and corpus striatum, autonomic ganglia, gastric and salivary gland and enteric nerves.
- **Receptor type**— G-protein coupled receptor (GPCR).

Mechanism of Action

The muscarinic receptors are G-protein coupled receptor (GPCR) having characteristic membrane domains. The M_1 and M_3 subtypes function through Gq protein and activate membrane bound phospholipase C (PLC); generating inositol triphosphate (IP_3) and diacylglycerol (DAG) which in turn release Ca^{+2} intracellularly, causing depolarization, glandular secretion and raise smooth muscle tone.

Functional Response

1. Increase in cognitive function (learning and memory)
2. Increase in seizure activity
3. Decrease in dopamine release and locomotion
4. Increase in depolarization of autonomic ganglia
5. Increase in secretions.

M_2 Receptors

Main Locations

Widely expressed in CNS and heart, also in visceral smooth muscle and autonomic nerve terminals.

Receptor Type

G-protein Coupled Receptor (GPCR)
Mechanism of action: The M_2 and M_4 receptor opens k^+ channels (through βγ subunits of regulatory protein Gi) and inhibits adenylyl cyclase (through α subunit of Gi) resulting in hyperpolarization, decrease in pacemaker

activity, slowing of conduction and decreased force of contraction in heart. Increased production of cyclic guanosine monophosphate (cGMP) and release of eicosanoids can also occur in certain tissues by activation of muscarinic receptors.

Functional Response
- *Heart*: Sinoatrial node (SA) node → slowed spontaneous depolarization and hyperpolarization, decrease in heart rate (HR). Atrioventricular node (AV node) → decrease in conduction velocity, atrium → decrease in refractory period, decrease in contraction.
- *Smooth muscles*: Increase in contraction.
- *Peripheral nerves*: Neural inhibition and decrease in ganglionic transmission.
- *Central nervous system (CNS)*: Neural inhibition, increase in tremor, hypothermia and analgesia.

M_3 Receptors

Site of Location

Widely expressed in CNS, abundant in smooth muscles and glands, vascular endothelium, iris, and ciliary muscle.

Mechanism of Action and Receptor as M_1

Functional response—gastric and salivary secretion, GI smooth muscle contraction, vasodilation, ocular accommodation, increase in body weight, fat deposits, increase in food intake, and inhibition of dopamine release.

M_4 Receptors

Site of Location

Vagal nerve endings, CNS—cortex and hippocampus, striatum.

MOA and Receptor

As M_2.

Action

Increase in locomotion, facilitation of dopamine release.

M_5 Receptors

Site of Location

Central nervous system (CNS), substantia nigra [Mechanism of action (MOA) as M_3], vascular endothelium of cerebral vessels.

Action

Dilatation of cerebral arteries and arterioles, facilitates dopamine release, augmentation of drug seeking behavior and reward.

ION CHANNEL RECEPTORS

These cell surface receptors enclose ion selective channels (for Na^+, K^+, Ca^{+2} and Cl^-) within their molecules. Agonist binding opens the channel and causes depolarization/hyperpolarization/changes in cytosolic ionic composition depending on the ion that flows through.

Examples of ion channel receptors are nicotinic cholinergic receptors, $GABA_A$ receptor, glycine receptors, NMDA (n methyl D-aspartate), $5HT_3$ receptors.

The receptor is usually a pentameric protein. In addition to the intra- and extracellular segments, the receptor has four membrane spanning domains, in each of which, amino acids (AA) chain traverses the width of the membrane six times. The subunits are arranged round the channel like a rosette and the α-subunits usually bear the agonist binding sites.

These are fast channels and takes milliseconds to produce action. The subunits are $α_2$, β, γ, δ each with molecular weight of 40–58 kDa. The four subunits show marked sequence homology and analysis of the hydrophobicity profile. The acetylcholine (ACh) binding site lie at the interface between one of the two α-subunits and its neighbor. Both must bind ACh molecules in order to be activated.

Nicotinic Receptor

Most excitatory neurotransmitters, such as acetylcholine (ACh) at the neuromuscular (NM) junction or glutamate in the central nervous system (CNS), cause an increase in Na^+ and K^+ permeability. This results in net inward current carried mainly by Na^+, which depolarizes the cell and increases the probability that it will generate action potential (AP).

The action can be indirect involving a G-protein and other intermediaries or direct, where the drug itself binds to the channel protein and alters its function, e.g. local anesthetics (LA) act on voltage gated Na^+ channels, drug molecule plugs the channel physically blocking ion permeation.

Example are:
- Dihydropyridines inhibit L-type calcium channel.
- Benzodiazepines bind to GABA receptor/chloride channel.
- Sulfonylureas act on adenosine triphosphate (ATP) sensitive potassium channels of β cells of pancreas.

Nonreceptor-mediated Drug Action

Drugs may target enzymes to produce their action. They may affect carriers or reuptake mechanisms for their actions. Cellular proteins like tubulin or immunophilines may also be targets for drug action.

Nicotinic Cholinergic Receptors (Fig. 1.6)

These receptors are selectively activated by nicotine and blocked by tubocurarine and hexamethonium. These are rosette-like pentameric structures which enclose a ligand gated cation channel. Activation of the channel

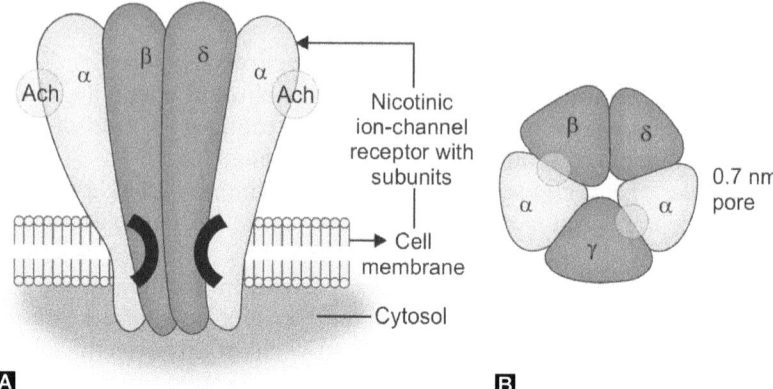

Figures 1.6A and B: Nicotinic acetylcholine receptor. (A) Longitudinal view; (B) Cross-sectional view.

causes opening of the channel with rapid flow of cations resulting in depolarization and generation of action potential. On the basis of location and selective agonists and antagonists two subtypes Nm and Nn are recognized.

Sites of Location

a. Muscle receptors which are confined to the skeletal neuromuscular junction.
b. Ganglionic receptors—sympathetic and parasympathetic ganglia.
c. CNS type receptors—brain.

Muscle Type (Nm) Receptor

$(\alpha 1)_2 \beta_1 \epsilon \delta$—Adult, $(\alpha 1)_2 \beta_1 \gamma \delta$—Fetal.
- *Site*: Skeletal neuromuscular junction.
- *Mechanism*: Opening of channel → increase in permeability of Na^+ and K^+. Excitatory end plate potential → depolarization → skeletal muscle contraction.
- *Agonists*: Acetylcholine (ACh), nicotine.
- *Antagonist*: Atracurium, vecuronium, d-tubocurarine and pancuronium.

Nn Type $(\alpha_3)_2 (\beta_4)_3$

- *Location*: Autonomic ganglia and adrenal medulla.
- *MOA*: Same—depolarization – secretion of catecholamines.
- *Agonist*: ACh and nicotine.
- *Antagonist*: Trimethaphan and mecamylamine.

CNS Type $(\alpha_4)_2, (\beta_4)_3, (\alpha_7)_5$

α-toxin Insensitive, α-toxin Sensitive

- *Location*: Pre- and postsynaptic.
- *MOA*: Same as in α-toxin sensitive channel which increases Ca^{+2} permeability.

- *Agonist*: Anatoxin A.
- *Antagonist*: Dihydro-β-erythrodine, mecamylamine for α-toxin insensitive; α-bungarotoxin, α-lonotoxin for α-toxin sensitive.

BIOTRANSFORMATION

Process by which the body brings about chemical changes in drug molecule is called biotransformation. It is needed to render nonpolar, lipid-soluble compounds more polar or lipid-insolubles, so that they are not reabsorbed in the renal tubules and are excreted. Most hydrophilic drugs, e.g. streptomycin, neostigmine, decamethonium, etc. are not biotransformed and are excreted unchanged. So, biotransformation reactions alter the physiochemical properties of a drug so that a drug with high lipid or water partition coefficient will be converted into a polar and water-soluble one for easy disposal from the body.

Organs Involved

Liver is the main organ involved. Other sites are intestinal mucosa, nasal epithelium, lungs, skin, (as cortisol, testosterone, betamethasone), kidney, (as insulin, vitamin D), brain (e.g. levodopa), plasma (e.g. succinylcholine, procaine).

Enzymes Involved

Microsomal

- These enzymes are present in the smooth endoplasmic reticulum (ER) of liver, kidneys and gastrointestinal tract (GIT). Important microsomal enzymes present in the hepatic cells are mixed function oxidase P450. Other enzymes are hydroxylase, reductase, dehydrogenase, glucuronyl transferase, glutathione S-transferase.

  The micorosomal enzymes are responsible for most of the oxidation reactions, some reduction, hydrolysis, glucuronidation and glutathione conjugation reactions. These enzymes are primarily the substrates of high lipid water partition coefficient. The microsomal enzymes can be inducible by drugs, diet and other factors.

Nonmicrosomal

- They are present in the cytoplasm, mitochondria and extracellular spaces of different organs. High concentration are found in the liver, plasma, kidneys and other tissues.

  Nonmicrosomal enzymes are esterase, amidase, hydrolase, sulfotransferase and glutathione S-transferase.

  These enzymes catalyze all conjugation reactions (except glucuronide and glutathione conjugation), hydrolysis, some oxidation and reduction reactions.

  These enzymes cannot be induced but can be inhibited by drugs.

Types

The chemical reactions involved in biotransformations are classified as—

Phase I Reactions

In which enzymes carry out oxidation, reduction on hydrolysis reactions. Phase I enzymes lead to the introduction of what are called functional groups, resulting in a modification of the drug, such that it now carries an OH, -COOH, -5H, -O, or NH_2 group. Reactions in phase I lead to inactivation of an active drug. In certain instances metabolism specially, hydrolysis of ester or amide linkage results in bioactivation of a drug which are called prodrugs. If the phase I metabolite is sufficiently polar, then it will be excreted in the urine. Some metabolites not excreted are further metabolized by phase II reactions. A single drug may undergo several biotransformation steps. Phase I oxygenases are—cytochrome P450 s, flavin containing monooxygenases (FMOs), epoxide hydrolases (MEH, SEH). The CYPs and FMOs are super families of enzymes. Each super family comprises multiple genes.

Cytochrome P450: Cytochrome P450 enzymes are heme proteins, comprising a large family (super family) of related but distinct enzymes (each referred to as CYP followed by a defining set of numbers and letters, number designates family and letter denoting the sub family). The name cytochrome P450 (CYP) is due the spectral properties of the hemoprotein. In its ferous form, it binds to carbon monoxide to produce a complex which absorbs maximum light at the range of 450 nm. These enzymes differ from one another in—
- Amino acid sequence.
- In regulation by inhibitors and inducing agents.
- In the specificity of the reactions they catalyze.

Different members of the family have distinct but often overlapping substrate specificities. This unusual feature of extensive overlapping substrate specificities by the CYPs is one of the underlying reasons for the predominance of drug-drug interactions.

Purification of P450 enzymes and DNA cloning has yielded 74 CYP gene families of which 3 main ones CYP1, CYP2, CYP3 are involved in drug metabolism in human liver. CYPIA2 is one of the main enzymes.

Heme contains one atom of iron in a hydrocarbon cage that functions to bind oxygen in the CYP active site as part of the catalytic cycle of these enzymes. CYPs use O_2 plus H^+ derived from the cofactor reduced nicotamide adenine dinucleotide phosphate (NADPH) to carry out the oxidation of substrates. The H^+ is supplied through the enzyme NADPH cytochrome P450 oxidoreductase. Metabolism of a substrate by a CYP consumes one molecule of molecular oxygen and produces an oxidized substrate and a molecule of water as a by product. The O_2 is usually converted to water by the enzyme superoxide dismutase.

The reactions carried out by mammalian CYPs are—
N - dealkylation, O - dealkylation aromatic hydroxylation, N - oxidation, S - oxidation deamination dehalogenation.

Inducers of P450	Inhibitors of P450
Rifampicin	Quinidine
Ethanol	Ketaconazole
Carbamazepine	Cimetidine
Phenobarbitone	Metronidazole
Glucocorticoids	Disulfiram
INH	Omeprazole
Chloral hydrate	Allopurinol
Phenylbutazone	Erythromycin
Griseofulvin	Clarithromycin
DDT	Chloramphenicol

As a family of enzymes CYPs are involved in the metabolism of dietary and xenobiotic agents, as well as synthesis of steroids and metabolism of bile acids. In contrast to the drug metabolizing CYPs, the CYPs that catalyze steroid and bile acid synthesis are substrate specific. The CYPs that carry out xenobiotic metabolism have a tremendous capacity to metabolize a large number of structurally diverse chemicals. The most active CYPs for drug metabolism are those in CYP2C, CYP2D, CYP3A subfamilies. CYP3A4 is the most abundantly expressed and involved in the metabolism of about 50% of clinically used drugs. Some examples—

- CYP1A1: Theophylline.
- CYP1A2: Caffeine, paracetamol, tacrine and theophylline.
- CYP2A6: Methoxyflurane.
- CYP2C9: Ibuprofen, phenytoxin, warfarin and tolbutamide.
- CYP2C19: Omeprazole.
- CYP2D6: Clozapine, codeine and metaprolol.
- CYP3A4/5: Cyclosporine, losartan, nifedipine and terfenadine.

Within human populations there are major sources of interindividual variation in CYP 450 enzymes. The causes include—genetic polymorphism, environmental factors, enzyme inhibitors and inducers, their presence in diet, e.g. grape fruit juice and St. John's wort (in alternative medicine) inhibit enzymes but Brussels sprout and cigarette smoke induce CYP 450 enzymes.

(Possible uses of enzyme induction—(1) congenital nonhemolytic jaundice—phenobarbitone, (2) Cushing's syndrome—phenytoin decreases manifestations, (3) liver disease and (4) chronic poisoning.)

Phase II (Conjugation) Reaction

If a drug molecule has a suitable hydroxyl, thiol or amino group, it is susceptible to conjugation reaction. The resulting conjugate is almost always pharmacologically inactive and less lipid soluble than its precursor and is excreted in urine or bile.

Conjugation with glucuronic acid, glycine conjugation, methylation, acetylation and sulfate occurs in phase II reactions.

SECOND MESSENGERS

As first messenger binds with its specific receptor, the drug receptor complex is formed which subsequently causes the synthesis and release of another intracellular regulatory molecule termed second messenger. These are— cyclic AMP, cyclic GMP, calcium, inositol 1, 4, 5 triphosphate, diacylglycerol, calmodulin.

Function

Second messenger molecules are produced in response to neurotransmitter binding to a receptor, translate the extracellular signal into a response that may be further propagated or amplified within the cell.
- Cyclic AMP—
  - First to be recognized.
  - Synthesized by plasma membrane attached adenylyl cyclase. Adenylyl cyclase converts adenosine triphosphate (ATP) into cyclic adenosine monophosphate (AMP).
  - Mediates responses, such as ionotropy, chronotropy of heart muscles, relaxation of smooth muscles, breakdown of carbohydrates in liver, breakdown of triglycerides (TG) in fat cells, calcium homeostasis, other endocrine and neural processes, acts exclusively through cyclic AMP dependent protein kinase (A kinase), phosphorylates enzymes and proteins involved in cell function-transfer of phosphate from ATP occurs.
- Calcium—intracellular calcium plays an important role in the function of most of the cells.
  - Intracellular calcium occurs in both bound and free form.
  - Free form of calcium is responsible for action.
  - Intracellular free calcium is about 10,000 times less compared to extracellular.
  - As cells are stimulated by agonist, intracellular Ca^{+2} concentration increases rapidly.
  - Intracellular free calcium brings about cellular action while bound form is present in the inner surface of cell membrane, ER, mitochondria, and secretory granules.
  - Responsible for neurotransmitter release, muscle contraction and various function.
- Cyclic GMP—
  - Cyclic GMP is produced from the guanosine triphosphate (GTP) by an enzyme guanylyl cyclase which is present in the inner phase of the plasma membrane.

- The enzyme is activated when muscarinic receptors are occupied by an agonist.
- Cyclic GMP → activates cyclic GMP-dependent protein kinase (G kinase).
- Subsequent effect is not yet known.
- Inositol 1, 4, 5 triphosphate—
  - Hydrolytic product of phosphatidyl (PI) inositol, a minor phospholipid of the cell membrane.
  - Activation of enzyme phospholipase which causes hydrolysis of phosphatidylinositol 4, 5 biphosphate (PIP_2).
  - Formation of water-soluble IP_3 and diacylglycerol.
  - This IP_3 stimulates release of Ca from ER, this Ca is responsible for effect.
  - IP_3 is then converted to IP_2, IP_1 inositol and finally PI.
- Diacylglycerol—
  - It formed from the metabolic product of PIP_2.
  - This diacylglycerol activates directly intracellular located protein kinase C (C kinase).
- Calmodulin—
  - Single peptide chain containing 148 amino acid residues.
  - Considered to be the receptor for intracellular free calcium.
  - It has four binding sites.
  - Three or four of these need to be occupied by Ca^{+2} before calmodulin will activate the myosin light chain kinase (MLCK)
  - As phosphorylated myosin forms cross bridges with actin and sliding of actin over myosin filaments occur—producing contraction of muscle.

ADVERSE DRUG REACTIONS

An adverse drug reaction may be defined as a harmful or significant effect caused by a drug at doses intended for therapeutic effect that warrants reduction of dose or withdrawal of the drug and foretells hazards from future administration. Adverse effect or reaction refer to all unwanted effects attributable to the drug.

All drugs are xenobiotics and there is nothing like a safe drug. Whenever a drug is administered a risk is undertaken. This risk may be due to the properties of the drug, patient factors of the environment.

Classification

Adverse drug reactions may be classified as—
- Type A or predictable reactions—based on the pharmacological properties which are "augmented". Effect often is reversible.
- Type B or unpredictable reactions—unrelated to pharmacological actions, e.g. idiosyncratic reactions. These effects are usually irreversible and bizarre. Such indirect toxicity may be direct or immunologic in nature, e.g. agranulocytosis with carbimazole. Other effects are liver or kidney

damage, bone marrow suppression, carcinogenesis and disordered fetal development.

According to cause adverse drug reactions may be classified as—
- *Side effects*: Unwanted often unavoidable pharmacodynamic effects that often occur at therapeutic doses.
- *Secondary effects*: These are indirect consequences of primary actions of the drug.
- *Toxic effects*: These are the result of excessive pharmacological actions of the drug due to either overdosage or due to prolonged or chronic use. The CNS, CVS kidney, liver, lung, skin and blood toxin organs are most commonly affected.
- *Drug-drug interactions*: With the use of polypharmacy, response of one drug may be altered due to the administration of another resulting in untoward effects.
- *Allergic drug reactions*: These are common form of adverse drug reactions. A drug or its metabolite can act as a hapten and can be immunogenic.

Type A Reactions

Over expression of normal pharmacological action, e.g.
- α_1 antagonists—causes hypotension.
- Anticoagulants—causes bleeding.
- Glycosides—causes cardiac arrhythmia.
- Anxiolytic—causes sedation.
- Insulin—causes hypoglycemia.

Type B Reactions

Rare and unpredictable, e.g.
- Paracetamol—causes hepatotoxicity.
- Thalidomide—causes teratogenicity.
- Chloramphenicol—causes aplastic anemia.
- Practalol—causes mucocutaneous syndrome.
- Carbimazole—causes agranulocytosis.

Side Effects

Unwanted effects due to pharmacodynamic profile of the drug in therapeutic dose regimens, e.g.
- Promethazine—causes sedation.
- Codeine—causes constipation.
- ACEI—causes cough.

Secondary Effects

Indirect consequences of primary action of the drug, e.g.
- Corticosteroids—causes osteoporosis.
- Tetracycline—causes superinfection.

Toxic Effects

Due to excessive pharmacological actions or due to direct tissue injury. Drug-induced cell damage occurs due to—

Noncovalent reactions: Lipid peroxidation, generation of toxic oxygen radicals, reactions causing depletion of glutathione, modification of sulfhydryl groups.

Covalent reactions: Targets are DNA and protein or peptide molecules, e.g.
- *Hepatotoxicity* — Paracetamol
  — INH
  — Iproniazid
  — Halothane
  — Methotrexate.

It occurs when hepatocytes are exposed to toxic metabolites from oxidation by CYP 450.

- *Nephrotoxicity*: Kidney is exposed to high concentration of drugs and drug metabolites. Renal damage occurs due to—interstitial nephritis, papillary or tubular necrosis, decrease in compensatory vasodilator PGs.

  Drug-induced nephrotoxicity occurs due to NSAIDs specially phenacetin ACE - I, methicillin, caffeine, captopril, cyclosporine.

- *Mutagenesis*: Mutation is a change in the genotype of a cell that is passed on when the cell divides. Chemical agents cause mutation by covalent modification of DNA. Mutation in protooncogenes, tumor suppressor genes result in carcinogenesis and usually involves more than one mutation. Drugs are relatively uncommon causes of birth defects and cancers.

- *Carcinogenesis*: Alteration of DNA is the first step in the complex multistage process of carcinogenesis. Carcinogens are chemical substances that cause cancer and can interact directly with DNA or act at a later stage to increase the likelihood that mutation will result in the production of a tumor. Most chemical carcinogens act by modifying bases in DNA particularly guanine, the O6 and N7 positions of which readily combine covalently with reactive metabolites of chemical carcinogens. Some therapeutic agents increase the risk of cancer—estrogen, pyrimethamine and methoxsalen.

- *Teratogenesis*: The term teratogenesis signifies production of gross structural malformations during fetal development. The timing of the teratogenic insult in relation to the stage of fetal development is critical in determining the type and extent of damage produced. It is during organogenesis days (17-60) that drugs can cause gross malformations. The structural organization of the embryo occurs in a well defined sequence, i.e. eye and brain, skeleton and limbs, heart and major blood vessels, palate and genitourinary system. The type of malformation produced thus depends on the time of exposure to the teratogen.

  Drugs with teratogenic potential are thalidomide, hydantoin, alcohol, nicotine, antithyroid drugs and steroids (stilbestrol).

Allergic Reaction to Drugs

It is the most common form of adverse responses to drugs. Most drugs being low molecular weight substances are not immunogenic in themselves. A drug or its metabolites act as a hapten by interacting with protein to form a stable conjugate that is immunogenic.

Drug-induced allergic reactions may be Ab-mediated (types I, II, III) or cell-mediated (type IV). Important clinical manifestations include—

- *Anaphylactic shock*: It may be life threatening due to respiratory obstruction. Most deaths are caused by penicillin. Drugs causing anaphylaxis are penicillin, streptokinase, asparginase, hormones, like ACTH, heparin, dextran, radiological contrast agents and vaccines.
  Treatment is done with injection of adrenaline which is lifesaving. Penicilloyl polylysine is used as a skin test reagent for penicillin allergy. Other type I reactions are—bronchospasm and urticaria.
- Drug-induced hematological reactions are produced by type II, type III, type IV hypersensitivity.
  - Type II reactions can affect any or all of the formed elements of the blood. Hemolytic anemia is related with sulfonamides and methyldopa.
  - Agranulocytosis which can be irreversible is caused by sulfonamides, chloramphenicol and carbimazole.
  - Thrombocytopenia is caused by quinine, heparin and thiazide diuretics.

Adverse Effects due to Chronic Use

- Eye—
  - Cataract—may be caused by chloroquine, steroids, phenothiazine and anticancer drugs.
  - Corneal opacity—may be caused by chloroquine, phenothiazine and amiodarone.
  - Retinal injury—may be caused by chloroquine, ethambutol and thioridazine.
- *Kidney*: Analgesic nephropathy caused by NSAIDs.
- *Allergic liver damage*: Type II, III—hypersensitivity reaction as in halothane hepatitis due to reactive metabolite of halothane which couples to liver protein to form an immunogen. Enflurane (trifluoroacetyl chloride) may also cause Ab—mediated liver damage.
- *Drug-induced SLE*: Type III reaction which involves antibody to nuclear material and is a multisystem disorder affecting skin, lung, kidney, CNS. Subsides when offending drug is stopped of hydralazine and procainamide.

Adverse Drug Reaction

Adverse drug reaction (ADR) is a major consequence of pharmacotherapy and monitoring is an integral part of good clinical practice. If adverse drug reactions are not noticed, unnecessary morbidity and mortality occurs, hence comes the importance of pharmacovigilance.

Prevention
- Easy availability of 'over the counter' drugs to be stopped.
- Genetic screening for status of GL-6-PO_4 dehydrogenase, pseudocholinesterase deficiency, acetylator status to be noted.
- Knowledge of the drug prescribed.
- Polypharmacy to be restricted to minimize drug-drug interactions.
- Recognition and reporting system of ADR to be practiced.
- Good clinical practices with detection of toxicities during preclinical as well as clinical trials.
- Finally risk-benefit ratio to be weighed before initiation of therapy.

CHAPTER 2

General Anesthetics

INTRODUCTION

- General anesthetics (GAs) are agents, which depress the central nervous system (CNS) to a sufficient degree to permit the performance of a surgery or other noxious or unpleasant procedures.
- GAs have low therapeutic indices.
- All GAs have similar actions but produce dissimilar side effects (S/E) on other organs.

HISTORY

- Ether was the first ideal anesthetic.
- Ether anesthesia was first used in 1842 by Crawford Long; first demonstration of GA was done by William TG Morton.
- Then came N_2O, used first by Horace Wells, a dentist, in 1845.
- James Simpson introduced chloroform in 1847; came into disuse due to its hepatotoxicity and cardiodepressant action.
- Cyclopropane came into use in 1929.
- Cyclopropane is explosive when mixed with air, O_2 or N_2O.
- Lundy demonstrated the use of thiopentone in 1935.
- Further development of other IV anesthetic agents led to total intravenous anesthesia (TIVA) use.

PHYSIOLOGICAL EFFECTS OF GENERAL ANESTHETICS

- *Cardiovascular system (CVS)*: Decrease in systemic arterial BP, direct vasodilation, myocardial depression, blunting of baroreceptor control, also decrease in central sympathetic tone.
    - Effects vary due to different agents and depend on the volume status and myocardial function of the patient.
- *Respiratory system*: GA decreases both ventilatory drive and the reflexes that maintain airway patency.

- Gag reflex and cough reflex are blunted.
- Lower esophageal sphincter (LES) tone is decreased, chance of regurgitation.
- *Hypothermia*: Patients tend to develop hypothermia (body temp. < 36°C) due to IV fluids, exposed body cavities and altered thermoregulatory control and decreased metabolic rate.
- Nausea and vomiting in the postoperative period due to action of GA on chemoreceptor trigger zone (CTZ) and brainstem vomiting center. So, $5HT_3$ antagonists like ondansetron is effective in suppressing the vomiting.
- Emergence and postoperative phenomenon may include the following:
  - Hypertension and tachycardia.
  - Myocardial ischemia may worsen in ischemic heart disease patients.
  - Neurological signs and symptoms, including delirium, spasticity and hyperreflexia.
  - Postanesthesia shivering.
  - Airway obstruction.
  - Pulmonary function is reduced.
  - Pain.

COMPONENTS OF GENERAL ANESTHESIA

- Amnesia.
- Immobility.
- Attenuation of autonomic responses to noxious stimuli.
- Analgesia.
- Unconsciousness.

Potency of a general anesthetic agent is usually measured by the minimum alveolar concentration (MAC).

MINIMUM ALVEOLAR CONCENTRATION

Definition

Minimum alveolar concentration values are generally quoted at steady conditions at 1 atmospheric pressure.

Inhalational agent	MAC (Vol %)
Halothane	0.75
Isoflurane	1.2
Enflurane	1.6
Sevoflurane	2
Desflurane	6
Nitrous oxide	105
Xenon	71

The MAC is defined as the minimum alveolar concentration that prevents movement in response to surgical stimulation in 50% of subjects. Lower the MAC value, more potent is the anesthetic agent.

Minimum alveolar concentration (MAC) (awake) when there is ability to respond to commands (verbal) and ability to form memories.

Standard noxious stimulus is the initial surgical skin incision. Response to stimulations must entail a positive gross purposeful muscular movement. Usually the head or extremities, coughing, rigidity, swallowing and chewing, even movement of an incised extremity, are not considered positive movement responses.

MAC concept has 4 basic components:
1. An all-none (quantal) movement response.
2. End-tidal concentration of anesthetic in alveoli.
3. Appropriate mathematical quantification of the relationship between points 1 and 2 mentioned above.
4. MAC can be quantitated for altered physiologic and pharmacologic states.

MAC can be evaluated as:
1. MAC—awake: Minimum alveolar concentration of anesthetic that would allow opening of the eyes on verbal command during emergence from anesthesia.
2. MAC—intubation: Minimum alveolar concentration of anesthetic that would inhibit movement and coughing during endotracheal intubation.
3. MAC—BAR: Minimum alveolar concentration of anesthetic necessary to prevent adrenergic response to skin incision.
4. MAC—skin incision: According to definition.

Utility of MAC

- MAC is an indication of drug concentration.
- MAC is dependent on barometric pressure.
- MAC of different inhalation agents can be compared.
- MAC is a sensitive tool to determine the interaction of other anesthetics and CNS drugs with inhaled anesthetics.
- MAC may be altered by various physiological and pharmacological states.

Factors Affecting MAC

- *Decrease in MAC*: Aging, narcotics, ketamine, benzodiazepines, barbiturates, IV local anesthetics, premedicants, N_2O, hypothyroidism (myxedema). Drugs which affect release of CNS neurotransmitter—reserpine, methyldopa, clonidine and pancuronium.
- *Increase in MAC*: Pyrexia, hyperthyroidism (thyrotoxicosis), alcoholism, sympathoadrenal stimulation, ephedrine, amphetamine and isoniazid (INH).
- *No effect*: Duration of anesthesia, sex and hyper/hypocarbia.

The MAC value is depicted under steady conditions of 1 atmospheric pressure. When more than one agent is used, their separate fractions may be added together to assess the total effect on the patient.

Factors Decrease MAC

1. Coadministration of other CNS depressant drugs, e.g. opioids, alcohol, sedatives.
2. Hypoxia, hypothermia and hypotension.
3. Old age.

MECHANISM OF ANESTHESIA

- Inhalational anesthetics can hyperpolarize neurons.
- May have substantial effects on synaptic transmission or propagation.
- A variety of ion channels, receptors and signal transduction proteins are modulated by general anesthetics, e.g. GABA-A, NMDA receptors and two pore potassium channels.
- Ketamine, N_2O and cyclopropane inhibit NMDA receptors.
- Halogenated inhalational anesthetics activate some members of a class of potassium channels.

GENERAL PRINCIPLES OF INHALATIONAL ANESTHESIA

Uptake of the anesthetic gas depends on:
- Partial pressure of the agent in the alveoli again depends on:
  - Concentration of the agent in the inspired gas.
  - Alveolar ventilation.
- Partial pressure of an anesthetic agent in the circulation again depends on:
  - Blood gas partition coefficient; ratio of concentration of the agent in the blood to that in gas in equilibrium.
  - Cardiac output or pulmonary blood flow.
  - Ventilation perfusion relationship.
- Partial pressure of an anesthetic agent in the brain/other tissues:
  - Cerebral blood flow.
  - Oil/gas partition coefficient ratio of the concentration of the agent in fat to that in gas. Hence is a measure of fat solubility.
  - Relative blood supply to different tissues.

The speed of equilibration of an anesthetic agent between the alveolar concentration and any tissue of the body depends upon a rich blood supply combined with a low agent solubility in the tissue.

CLINICAL SIGNS OF ANESTHESIA (BASED ON ETHER ANESTHESIA)

- Stage of analgesia:
  - Loss of eyelash reflex.
  - Other reflexes present.
  - Loss of consciousness.

- Stage of excitement:
  - Excitement and restlessness.
  - Irregular breathing.
  - Heart rate and BP may rise.
  - Regurgitation, coughing and laryngospasm may occur.
- Stage of surgical anesthesia:
  - Plane 1—Roving eyeballs → get fixed.
  - Plane 2—Loss of corneal and laryngeal reflexes.
  - Plane 3—Pupils begin dilating, loss of light reflex.
  - Plane 4—Intercostal paralysis, fully dilated pupil.
- Stage of medullary paralysis.

Elimination

- All inhalational agents are mostly eliminated via lungs. Anesthetics may remain for prolonged periods in the adipose tissue due to high lipid solubility of the agent and minimum blood supply of adipose tissue. Most GAs are eliminated unchanged by exhalation excepting halothane, 20% of which is metabolized in the liver.

COMMON ANESTHETICS

HALOTHANE

- 2 bromo-2 chloro-1, 1, 1-, trichloroethane.
- Potent, noninflammable and nonexplosive.
- Volatile liquid, decomposed by light hence stored in amber-colored bottles.
- Can be used safely with soda lime.
- As it is subject to spontaneous breakdown, it is marketed along with preservative thymol.
- Decomposed by an open flame and liberating bromine.
- High blood: Gas partition coefficient and high fat: blood partition coefficient.
- Induction, therefore is slow and smooth, remains in lipid-rich tissue for prolonged periods.
- 60-80% of halothane inhaled is eliminated unchanged by lungs in the first 24 hours after its administration.
- > 20% is metabolized by hepatic cytochromes P450 (CYPs).
- Major metabolite of halothane is trifluoroacetic acid, which is formed by removal of bromine and chlorine ions.
- Intermediate metabolite trifluoroacetylchloride can trifluoroacetylate several proteins in liver as immune reaction resulting in fulminant hepatic necrosis, though rarely seen.

Use—induction and maintenance of GA especially in pediatric group.
- Advantages—pleasant to inhale, smooth induction, potent and low cost.

Actions

CVS

- Myocardial depressant.
- Sinus/nodal bradycardia common due to increase in vagal tone.
- Dilation of coronary arteries.
- Increase in myocardial O_2 demand.
- Decrease in baroreceptor reflex (fails to correct negative inotropy and chronotropy).
- Hypotension arrhythmia can occur due to CO_2 retention.
- Sensory stimulation in light plane/or catecholamine release.

CNS

- Smooth and rapid induction.
- Moderate degree of muscle relaxation and potentiation of non-depolarizing muscle relaxant.
- Increase in cerebral blood flow and decrease in cerebral metabolism.
- Autoregulation of renal, splanchnic and cerebral blood flow is inhibited by halothane.

Respiratory System
- Rapid and shallow respiration.
- Elevation of arterial CO_2 tension.
- Effective bronchodilation.

Uterus
Uterine smooth muscle is relaxed, prolongs labor and can cause postpartum hemorrhage (PPH).

Temperature
Following induction, there may be drop of up to 1°C core temperature followed by rise of up to 4°C skin temperature. It can cause malignant hyperthermia.

Kidney
- Halothane—induce reduction in renal blood flow.
- Decrease in glomerular filtration rate (GFR).
- Hepatic and gastrointestinal (GI) tract— decrease hepatic and splanchnic blood flow—1 in 10,000 can suffer from halothane hepatitis.

Halothane hepatitis syndrome: It is characterized by fever, anorexia, nausea, vomiting occurring several days after anesthesia. It may be accompanied with rash and peripheral eosinophilia.

Metabolites are slowly cleared from the body for a period of 3 weeks. Hence, careful history of halothane exposure should be taken before administration—should not be used within 3 months of previous halothane anesthesia.

ISOFLURANE
- 1-chloro-2, 22-trifluoroethyl difluoromethyl ether.
- Volatile liquid and colorless with pungent odor.
- Neither inflammable nor explosive.
- Blood gas partition coefficient lower than halothane/enflurane.
- Induction and recovery with isoflurane is faster than that of halothane.
- Stable, so no preservative is required, does not react with metal or soda lime.

Actions

CVS
- Produces concentration-dependent decrease in arterial BP.
- Cardiac output is maintained.
- Vasodilation in most vascular beds especially skin and muscle.
- Increase in coronary blood flow and decrease in myocardial O_2 demand makes isoflurane ideal for patients with ischemic heart disease.
- Might produce 'coronary steal' phenomenon.
- Depresses baroreceptor reflexes.

Respiratory System
- Concentration-dependent decrease in respiration.
- Normal respiratory rate but decrease in tidal volume.
- Increase in CO_2 retention due to alveolar ventilation is decreased.
- Effective bronchodilation.
- Also irritant to the airway.

CNS
- Increased cerebral blood flow but vasodilation is less than halothane or enflurane.
- Decreased cerebral metabolism in dose-dependent manner reduces cerebral metabolic rate by 50%.

Muscle
- Relaxation of skeletal muscle.
- Potentiation of neuromuscular blocking agents.
- Also relaxes uterine smooth muscle.

Miscellaneous
Isoflurane has anticonvulsive properties and does not allow development of cerebral edema after trauma.

Kidney and Liver
- Decreased renal blood flow and decreased GFR.
- Hepatic portal blood flow is decreased but arterial blood flow maintained.

ENFLURANE
Similar to isoflurane, except:
- Epileptiform EEG changes can occur especially in hypercapnia.
- Convulsions can occur in patients who have history of epilepsy.
- Greater muscle relaxation compared with isoflurane.
- Poor analgesia.
- 2–8% of absorbed enflurane undergoes oxidative metabolism in liver.
- Patient on isoniazid (INH) therapy exhibits enhanced metabolism of enflurane with significant elevated serum fluoride concentration.
- Used for maintenance rather than induction like, isoflurane.

DESFLURANE
- Requires the use of a specially heated vaporizer because boiling point (BP) of desflurane is close to room temperature.
- Reacts with dry soda lime to produce carbon monoxide.
- Sympathetic hyperactivity can occur, myocardial sensitization to catecholamines does not occur, 'coronary steal' not reported.
- Irritant to airway; so intravenous induction agent is used.

- Suitable for day-care surgery due to extremely low blood gas partition coefficient. So, rapid induction and rapid recovery. Otherwise, similar to isoflurane.

SEVOFLURANE

- Can undergo an exothermic reaction with dessicated CO_2 absorbent (baralyme) to produce airway burn/spontaneous ignition or explosion.
- Can also produce CO with dessicated CO_2 absorbent.
- 3% of administered sevoflurane is biotransformed, predominant product being hexafluoroisopropanol.
- Heart rhythm is stable with no sensitization to catecholamines or any evidence of coronary steal.
- Used for rapid and smooth induction in both children and adults; but should not be used in a closed circuit.
- Suitable for day-care surgery.
- Interaction of sevoflurane with soda lime produces decomposition products, major product compound A is renotoxic.
- The Food and Drug Administration (FDA) recommends sevoflurane to be administered with fresh gas flows of at least 2 liters/minute to minimize accumulation of compound A.

NITROUS OXIDE

- Noninflammable and nonexplosive.
- Potent analgesic.
- Rapid induction and rapid recovery.
- Not a potent anesthetic and MAC 105.
- Second gas effect—serves to concentrate coadministered halogenated anesthetics.
- Diffusion hypoxia—during discontinuation N_2O can rapidly fill up the alveoli and diluting O_2 in the lung, thereby causing hypoxia.
- N_2O can oxidize the cobalt I (CO) form of vitamin B_{12} to CO_3, thereby preventing vitamin B_{12} from acting as a cofactor for methionine synthetase which is important in synthesis of DNA, RNA and myelin.
- Methionine synthetase activity becomes depressed after 3-4 hours of N_2O exposure and activity is restored in 3-4 days.
- May cause megaloblastic anemia and peripheral neuropathy.
- Cannot be used at concentration >80%.
  Will exchange with N_2 in any air-containing cavity in the body as N_2O will move faster than N_2 escapes; thereby increased the volume of pneumothorax, pulmonary or intestinal bullae or any enclosed air bubble.

Second Gas Effect

Under normal circumstances, only O_2 is taken up from the lungs and there is no net uptake of N_2O. As a second gas which is absorbed rapidly, N_2O is introduced into the lungs. Uptake of (N_2O) has the effect of concentrating other gases remaining in the alveoli, e.g. halothane. This is called second gas effect.

The effect on O_2 is of no clinical importance but the increase in concentration of volatile anesthetic agent like halothane speeds the induction of anesthesia.

The reverse occurs when administration of N_2O is stopped. The elimination of the gas (N_2O) dilutes the alveolar gases and results in significant hypoxemia unless FiO_2 is increased. This effect lasts for 5 minutes after discontinuation of N_2O.

Diffusion Hypoxia

As administration of N_2O is discontinued at the end of anesthesia, N_2O diffuses out of blood into the alveoli in larger volumes.

Consequently, the alveolar concentration of other gases, e.g. O_2 are diluted. Similarly PaO_2 is reduced and arterial oxygenation impaired if the patient breathes air. $PaCO_2$ is reduced also causing hypoventilation. SpO_2 is reduced below baseline to values as low as 90% for several minutes in normal individuals after breathing 50% N_2O in O_2. Arterial desaturation is greater in elderly patients if higher concentrations of N_2O have been used or if $PaCO_2$ is low initially because of hypoventilation.

So, at the end of anesthesia diffusion, hypoxia is avoided by the administration of O_2 for 10 minutes after discontinuation of N_2O anesthesia.

Diffusion hypoxia in healthy individual is usually transient and the extent of reduction in PaO_2 may be in the order 0.5-1.5 KPa.

Points to Note (Evidence-based)

- Nitrous oxide use is associated with postoperative nausea, vomiting, increased risk of postoperative complications like pneumonia and wound infection.
- Volatile anesthetics reduce the risk of MI and death in patients after coronary artery surgery compared with IV anesthetic.
- Halothane lacks the ether moiety, structurally present in isoflurane, sevoflurane and desflurane and this accounts for its propensity to cause ventricular cardiac dysrhythmia.
- Isoflurane and desflurane structurally differ in substitution of the one chlorine atom for fluorine, fluorine substitution renders greater stability and resistance to metabolism.

XENON

Xenon, an inert gas which cannot be manufactured but is extracted from air. Hence, it is expensive and available only in limited amount.

MAC Value 55-71

It has analgesic action, due to antagonism of NMDA receptors and agonism of TREK channel (member of two pore K^+ channel family).

Extremely insoluble in blood and produces rapid induction and emergence from anesthesia.

Can be used along with 30% oxygen to produce surgical anesthesia or as supplementation along with IV anesthetic agent.

Well tolerated with minimum cardiorespiratory adverse effects.

THERAPEUTIC GASES

Oxygen, carbon dioxide, nitric oxide, helium, hydrogen sulfide, etc.

Uses

Oxygen—to reverse or prevent hypoxia.
- Decreased ventilation.

Carbon dioxide—insufflation for endoscopic procedures, especially in abdominal laparoscopic surgeries.
- Cardiac surgery and cardiopulmonary bypass surgery.

Nitric oxide—inhaled nitric oxide is FDA approved for treatment of persistent pulmonary hypertension as it selectively dilates pulmonary vasculature.
- Diagnostic use during cardiac catheterization in patients with heart failure and infants with congenital heart disease.
- For measurement of fractional exhaled NO, as a noninvasive marker of airway inflammation and assessment of respiratory tract disease.

Helium—noble gas with characteristic physical and chemical properties, making it useful for medical use.

It is inert, with low density, low solubility and high thermal conductivity and has wide variety of uses.
- Helium and oxygen mixture (79/21) has light weight and is used for improving flow of oxygen in upper airway obstruction and asthma exacerbation.
- Helium and oxygen mixture (Heliox), rather than nitrous oxide is preferred to prevent nitrogen bubbles.
- In pulmonary MRI radiology and imaging of organs (using helium ion microscopy).
- Use of helium in insufflation during abdominal laparoscopy.
- Assessment of pulmonary function.
- Myocardial protection from ischemia.
- Neuroprotective to brain.
- During laser airway surgery.
- As adjunct therapy in COPD, asthma, ARDS, and bronchiolitis.

Hydrogen sulfide—colorless, inflammable, water-soluble gas with characteristic rotten egg smell.
- Activates ATP dependent K^+ channels and has vasodilating properties.
- Serves as a free radical scavenger and has potential to limit cell death.
- Protects body against damage due to hypoxia, hemorrhage, ischemia or reperfusion injury.

CHAPTER 3

Parenteral Anesthetics

INTRODUCTION

Intravenous anesthetic agents are:
- Small, hydrophobic aromatic/heterocyclic compounds.
- Due to hydrophobicity, they preferably partition into highly perfused and lipophilic tissue, e.g. brain.
- Drug redistribution occurs; may remain stored in lipid-rich tissues.
- Half-life varies from drug to drug.

IDEAL ANESTHETIC (IV) AGENT

- Highly lipid-soluble and pH that of plasma.
- Highly unionized at plasma pH.
- Cheap, easily available.
- Long shelf-life, no mixing and diluting or preservation should be necessary.
- Rapid onset and recovery.
- No active metabolites.
- Good analgesic.
- Should not release histamine.
- No excitatory phenomenon.
- High therapeutic index.
- Should not produce pain on injection.
- Should not have untoward central nervous system (CNS), cardiovascular system (CVS) and respiratory effects.
- No important drug interactions.

Comparison of different IV anesthetics is listed in Table 3.1 whereas comparative study of pharmacodynamic parameters of some anesthetic agents are given in Table 3.2. On the other hand, doses and precautions of some IV anesthetic agents are listed in Table 3.3.

Table 3.1: Comparison of IV anesthetics.

Drug and its pH	Formulation	IV dose	Induction dose duration	Protein binding
Thiopentone pH 10–11	25 mg/mL in aqueous solution + 1.5 mg/mL Na_2CO_3	3–5 mg/kg	5–8 minutes	85%
Methohexital pH 10–11	10 mg/mL in solution + 1.5 mg/mL Na_2CO_3	1–2 mg/kg	4–7 minutes	85%
Propofol pH 4.5–7	10 mg/mL in 10% soybean oil, 2.25% glycerol, 1.2%, egg phosphatide, EDTA, etc.	1.5–2.5 mg/kg	4–8 minutes	98%
Etomidate pH 6.9	2 mg/mL in 35% propylene glycol	0.2–0.4 mg/kg	4–8 minutes	76%
Ketamine pH 3.5–5.5	10/50/100 mg/mL in aqueous solution	0.5–1.5 mg/kg	10–15 minutes	27%

BARBITURATES

- Derivatives of barbituric acid.
- The 3 barbiturates commonly used in clinical anesthesia are thiopentone sodium, thiamylal and methohexital.
- Supplied as racemic mixtures.
- Formulated as sodium salts with 6% Na_2CO_3.
- To be reconstituted in water/isotonic saline to produce 2.5% thiopental, 2% thiamylal and 1% methohexital.
- Solutions are highly alkaline (pH 10-11).
- Induction dose of thiopentone is 3-4 mg/kg with onset of action in 10-30 second; peak effect 1 minute and duration of action 5-8 minutes.
- Neonates require higher dose while elderly and pregnant people require less; dose can also be reduced when premedication with opiates, benzodiazepines or α_2-adrenergic agonists are given.
- Thiopentone is most commonly used as inducing agent while thiamylal is used only for veterinary use.
- Methohexital is 3-fold more potent than thiopentone (onset of action and duration similar) while thiamylal is equipotent.
- Redistribution effect limits its duration of action.
- Prolonged infusions may result in accumulation of drug.
- Methohexital differs from other two, due to its rapid clearance and less accumulation.
- Psychomotor impairment may last up to 8 hours.
- Hepatic metabolism and renal excretion of inactive metabolites; a fraction of thiopental is desulfurated to the longer acting pentobarbital.
- Highly protein bound.

CNS
- Decrease in cerebral metabolic rate in a dose-dependent ratio can be used as protectant against cerebral ischemia.
- Reduces intraocular pressure and anticonvulsant.

CVS
- Dose-dependent decrease in BP due to venodilation and decrease in myocardial contractility.
- Myocardial O_2 supply: Demand ratio is maintained.
- Compensatory tachycardia may be nominal due to blunting of baroreceptor reflex.
- Hypotension is severe in patients with hypovolemia, cardiomyopathy and coronary artery disease.

Respiratory System
- Respiratory depression, decrease in minute volume, tidal volume (TV) and respiratory rate.
- Reflex response to hypercarbia and hypoxia are diminished.
- Higher incidence of wheezing in asthmatic patients due to release of histamine.
- Can induce fatal attacks of porphyria in patients with acute intermittent or variegate porphyria.
- Methohexital can produce pain on injection.
- Excitatory symptoms, e.g. cough, hiccup, tremor or twitching/hypertonus can be seen.

PROPOFOL
- 2, 6-di-isopropylphenol is an oil at room temperature and insoluble in aqueous solution.
- Formulated for IV administration as a 1% emulsion in 10% soybean oil, 2.25% glycerol and 1.2% purified egg phosphatide; disodium EDTA or sodium metabisulfite may be added to inhibit bacterial growth.
- Should be used within 4 hours. After removing it from sterile packaging.
- Emulsion formulation is associated with pain on injection; aqueous formulation, fospropofol is devoid of it.
- Fospropofol is a prodrug; it is hydrolized by endothelial alkaline phosphatases to yield propofol, phosphate and formaldehyde.
- Induction dose 2–2.5 mg/kg; onset and duration similar to thiopental; 10–50% of induction dose can be used every 5 minutes for maintenance of anesthesia; 100–300 µg/kg/min can be used in infusion pump.
- Onset of action within 10 minutes and duration about 45 minutes.
- Rapid clearance is responsible for shorter duration of action.
- Metabolized in the liver by conjugation to sulfate and glucuronide; excreted in urine.
- Highly protein bound.
- Half-life for hydrolysis of fospropofol is 8 minutes.

CNS
- Sedation and hypnosis occurs via $GABA_A$ receptors resulting in increase in chloride conduction and hyperpolarization of neurons.
- Propofol decrease in cerebral blood flow, intracranial and intraocular pressures.
- Similar neuroprotective as thiopentone; efficacy not yet established.

CVS
- Dose-dependent decrease in BP due to both vasodilaton and mild depression of myocardial contractility.
- Blunts the baroreceptor reflex and reduces sympathetic nerve activity.
- Should be used cautiously in hypovolemia; hypotension and significant blood loss (like thiopentone).

Respiratory System
- Respiratory depression more than thiopentone.
- Oxygenation and ventilation should be monitored.
- Does not cause bronchospasm.

Others
- No significant effects on liver, kidney or other endocrine organs.
- It has no antianalgesic action.
- It has antiemetic action.
- Rare but potentially fatal complication termed as propofol infusion syndrome can be seen in prolonged high-dose infusion of propofol. Syndrome is characterized by metabolic acidosis, hyperlipidemia, rhabdomyolysis and enlarged liver.

ETOMIDATE
- Substituted imidazole that is supplied as the active d-isomer.
- Poorly soluble in water; formulated in 35% propylene glycol.
- Primarily used for anesthetic induction of patients with risk for hypotension.
- Induction dose is 0.2–0.6 mg/kg; has a rapid onset and short duration of action.
- Accompanied by high incidence of pain on injection and myoclonic movements.
- May be given rectally; onset of action 5 minutes.
- Redistribution limits its duration of action.
- Metabolism primarily occurs in the liver; elimination occurs via the kidney (78%) and liver (22%).
- High plasma protein binding.

CNS
- Produces hypnosis.
- No analgesic action.
- Decreased cerebral blood flow (CBF), metabolism, intraocular and intracranial pressure.
- Used as a protectant against cerebral ischemia.

CVS
- Cardiovascular stability after induction is of major advantage.
- Small increase in heart rate but minimum or no decrease in blood pressure or cardiac output.
- Little effect on coronary perfusion pressure but decrease myocardial O_2 demand.
- Hence, IV agent of choice in ischemic heart disease (IHD), cardiomyopathy cerebrovascular disease or hypovolemia.

Respiratory System
- Degree of respiratory depression is less.
- Does not release histamine significantly.

Others
- Associated with nausea and vomiting.
- Mildly and transiently reduce cortisol. Recently an ultrashort-acting analogue, methoxy-carbonyl-etomidate has been developed that does not produced adrenocortical suppression.

KETAMINE
- Arylcyclohexylamine and a phencyclidine congener.
- Supplied as a mixture of R and S isomers though S-isomer is more potent with fewer side effects.
- Lipophilic, water-soluble; supplied in 10, 50, 100 mg/mL solution in NaCl with preservative benzethonium chloride.
- Produces rapid hypnosis, profound analgesia and amnesia with eyes open and limbs moving involuntarily under spontaneous breathing. This cataleptic state has been termed as dissociative anesthesia.
- Administered IV, IM orally and rectally.
- Induction dose 0.5–1 mg/kg IV; 4–6 mg/kg IM and 8–10 mg/kg rectally. For maintenance an infusion of 25–100 μg/kg/min may be used.
- Metabolized to norketamine which has reduced CNS activity; norketamine is further metabolized and excreted in urine and bile.
- Large volume of distribution.
- Less protein binding compared to other IV agents.

Table 3.2: Comparative study of pharmacodynamic parameters of some drug anesthetic agents.

Drug	CBF	CMR	ICP	MAP	HR	CO	RR
Thiopentone	↓	↓	↓	↓	↑	↓	↓
Propofol	↓	↓	↓	↓	↑	↓	↓
Etomidate	↓	↓	↓	0	0	0	0
Ketamine	↑	0	↑	↑	↑	↑	0

(CBF: Cerebral blood flow; CMR: Cerebral metabolic rate; ICP: Intracranial pressure; MAP: Mean arterial pressure; HR: Heart rate; CO: Cardic output; RR: Respiratory rate)

CNS

- Indirect sympathomimetic activity.
- Ketamine-induced cataleptic state is accompanied by nystagmus with pupillary dilation, salivation, lacrimation, spontaneous limb movements and increased muscle tone.
- Profound analgesia.
- Increased CBF, increased intraocular and intracranial tension.
- Emergence delirium characterized by hallucinations, vivid dreams and delusions.

CVS

- Increased BP, heart rate and CO.
- Arrhythmogenic.
- Increased myocardial O_2 demand.
- Not ideal for patients at risk of MI.

Respiratory System

- Small and transient decrease in minute ventilation.
- Potent bronchodilation.
- Increased secretions.

The main limitation of ketamine is its unpleasant psychomimetic adverse effects but its unique features of potent analgesia and minimal respiratory depression are of advantage. Most recently ketamine is used in subanalgesic doses to limit or reverse opioid tolerance.

Parenteral anesthetics are the most common drugs used in induction of anesthesia.

Reasons for using an inducing agent:
- Quick onset and short duration of action.
- Lipophilicity.
- Relatively high perfusion in brain and spinal cord.
- May accumulate in fatty tissue prolonging recovery.
- Thiopentone and propofol are most commonly used.

- Etomidate is reserved for patients with hypotension and/myocardial ischemia.
- Ketamine is noteworthy for its strong analgesic action and preferred in patients with asthma or those undergoing short and painful procedures.

MIDAZOLAM

- Exists in two dynamic isomers; the open diazepine ring form is water-soluble but the closed ring form is not.
- Dose is 0.1–0.3 mg/kg for induction.
- Onset is slower and less predictable.
- Co-induction with a small IV dose (1–3 mg of midazolam) allows a reduction in the dose of propofol required.
- Can be administered via IV as well as nasal, oral, rectal routes as premedicant.
- Acts on γ-subunit of $GABA_A$ receptor domain and augments hyperpolarization by increase in the frequency of channel opening (thiopental, propofol, etomidate increase in the duration of channel opening).
- Actions may be reversed by flumazenil.
- *Central nervous system (CNS)*: Sedation, hypnosis, anticonvulsant, amnesia more than diazepam. More effective in terminating seizures in children.
- *Respiratory system*: Decrease in respiratory rate and depth, apnea can occur during induction.
- *Cardiovascular system (CVS)*: Stable, BP is maintained in low doses. Reflex tachycardia compensates for any fall.
- Hepatic metabolism by CYP3A4, CYP2A19, hydroxylated, glucuronidated and excreted via kidney.
- A state of confusion can occur on prolonged administration as in intensive therapy unit (ITU).

FENTANYL

- Short-acting potent opioid.
- Used to supplement balanced anesthesia.
- Permits the use of lower anesthetic concentration with better hemodynamic stability.
- Dose 2–4 µg/kg IV.
- Reflex effects of painful stimuli are abolished.
- Patient remains drowsy but his cooperation can be commanded.
- Vagal stimulation of heart results in decreased heart rate.
- Slight fall in BP (blood pressure).
- Nausea and vomiting during recovery.
- Increased tone of chest muscles (board-like rigidity) may follow rapid fentanyl infusion.
- Duration of action is about 30 minutes.
- Opioid antagonist naloxone may be used to treat persisting respiratory depression.

Table 3.3: Commonly used IV anesthetic agents with doses and precautions.

Drug; (Generic and trade name)	Dosage form	Induction dose	Infusion dose	Precautions
Propofol Propovan	10 mg/mL or 20 mg/mL vials	2 mg/kg	100–200 μg/kg/min for TIVA; 20–50 μg/kg/min for sedation	Produces dose-dependent respiratory depression
Ketamine Aneket Ketmin Ketamax Ketam	10 mg/mL in 10/20 mL vial, 50 mg/mL in 2 mL/10 mL vial	0.5–2 mg/kg IV, 3–10 mg/kg IM/oral/Rectal	5–20 μg/kg/min	Hallucinations, ↑ICT, ↑BP; do not coadminister salbutamol/aminophylline/magnesium
Midazolam Fulsed Mezolam Midosed	1 mg/mL in 5 mL/10 mL vials	0.2–0.3 mg/kg	0.02–0.1 mg/kg/hr	Hypotension may occur
Fentanyl Fendrop Fent Trofentyl	Injection 50 μg/mL in 2 mL ampoule, oral, sublingual tablets of 200/300/400 μg	2–4 μg/kg	1–5 μg/kg/hr	Risk of respiratory depression when coadministered with other sedatives

- Also used as adjunct in spinal, nerve block anesthesia and to relieve postoperative pain, cancer pain.
- Alfentanil, sufentanil, remifentanil are shorter acting analogues which can be used.

Droperidol

Derivative of haloperidol, when used in combination with fentanyl produces neuroleptanesthesia not used nowadays.

Nowadays droperidol is primarily used as antiemetic with sedative and antipruritic effect.

It should always be used under electrocardiogram (ECG) monitoring due to its potential for prolonging QT interval and producing fatal cardiac arrhythmias. Dose: 10–20 μg/kg.

TOTAL INTRAVENOUS ANESTHESIA (TIVA)

Definition: Complete provision of anesthesia (analgesia, unconsciousness and muscle relaxation) entirely by IV route.

Properties of drugs used in TIVA should ideally be as follows:
- Water-soluble: Thereby use of solvent is avoided.

- Stable in solution and on exposure to light.
- No absorption in plastic tubing.
- No venous damage or tissue damage.
- Sleep produced in one arm-brain circulation time.
- Short duration of action.
- Metabolism mainly in liver.
- Inactive, nontoxic, water-soluble metabolite.
- Minimum respiratory or circulatory side effect.

Indications

- As an alternative to volatile agent or to supplement O_2-N_2O.
- To provide sedation during regional technique.
- Ambulatory surgery where complete recovery is important.
- When N_2O is not desirable, e.g. one-lung anesthesia, middle ear surgery, neuroanesthesia, prolonged abdominal surgery, relief of cardiac disease, bronchoscopy and laryngoscopy.

Advantages

- In the doses required for TIVA, minimum cardiovascular depression occurs.
- Rapid recovery of consciousness.
- Good recovery of psychomotor function.
- Allows a high inspired concentration of O_2.
- Decrease in postoperative nausea and vomiting (PONV) and operation theater (OT) pollution.

Disadvantages

- Possibility of awareness.
- Likelihood of postoperative respiratory depression.
- Requirement of separate intravenous (IV) access site.
- Inability to control depth of anesthesia.

Techniques of Administration

a. *Intermittent injection*: Acceptable for procedures of short duration.
b. *Manual infusion technique*: Infusion rate in µg/min = steady state plasma concentration (kg/mL) × clearance (µg/mL/min). Fixed rate infusion is inappropriate because serum concentration of drug increases slowly by taking more time to reach steady state. A bolus dose followed by continuous infusion is preferable, e.g. propofol in bolus dose 1 mg/kg is followed by 10 mg/kg for 10 minutes, then 8 mg/kg for 10 minutes, then 6 mg/kg for next 10 minutes. Plasma concentration achieved is 3 µg/ml which is satisfactory in nonparalyzed patients.
c. *Computer-driven technique*: The drug is infused by a syringe driver which infuses the bolus dose rapidly followed by progressively decreasing infusion rate as programed in the computer.

Dexmedetomidine

- Active enantiomer of medetomidine.
- Centrally acting selective α_{2A}-agonist, useful in decreasing anesthetic requirement.
- Used as short-term sedative in intensive care unit (ICU) or as an adjunct in anesthesia.
- Provides sedation, anxiolysis, hypnosis, analgesia as well as sympatholysis. The sedative action of dexmedetomidine is unique because it resembles physiological sleep; acts through endogenous sleep pathways.

Advantage:
- Both analgesia and sedation are produced.
  - No respiratory depression
  - Obliteration of sympathetic reflexes.
- Adverse effects: Hypotension, nausea, dry mouth and bradycardia.
- Dose: 1 µg/kg given over 10 minutes as loading dose.
  - Infusion—0.2-0.7 µg/kg/hr
- Precautions: Hypovolemia and hypotension.
  - Does not produce amnesia, additional drug required.

CONSCIOUS SEDATION

A state of central nervous system (CNS) depression is produced so as to sedate the patient for minor therapeutic, diagnostic or dental procedures without altering consciousness. Undertaken in apprehensive patients or patients whose cooperation is required during such procedures. The protective airway reflexes are unaltered.

Drugs used for conscious sedation:
- Diazepam: 1-2 mg IV repeated hourly.
- Midazolam: 0.02-0.1 mg/kg/hr.
- Propofol: 25-50 µg/kg/min.
- Fentanyl: 1-2 µg/kg IV repeated at 30 minutes interval.
- Nitrous oxide: Along with O_2 in 10% increments to a maximum of 50%.

Similar to inhalational anesthetics, intravenous anesthetics too do not produce all the desired effects of hypnosis, amnesia, analgesia and immobility required for anesthesia. Hence, balanced anesthesia comprising smaller doses of multiple drugs including inhaled anesthetics, sedative hypnotics, opioid and neuromuscular blocking drugs, is practiced today.

ROLE OF α_2-RECEPTOR AGONISTS (CLONIDINE AND DEXMEDETOMIDINE) IN ANESTHESIA

- Clonidine and dexmedetomidine act by binding to presynaptic α_2 receptors and inhibit norepinephrine release.
- Produces analgesia, sedation, anxiolysis, hypotension and in large doses produces a state mimicking normal sleep.
- At the level of spinal cord, α_2 receptor stimulation helps in modulation of pain pathways producing analgesia.

- Moreover, there is decrease in peripheral vascular resistance, decrease in systemic BP and heart rate. However, in very high dose, they may act additionally on α_1-receptors, induce vasoconstriction, hence cause BP rise.

	Clonidine	Dexmedetomidine
Route	Oral, IV, IM, transdermal, transthecal, epidural	IV route only
Therapeutic index	Broad therapeutic index	Broader therapeutic index
Receptor affinity	High affinity for α_2 receptors	Higher affinity for α_2 receptors
Increase in dose	Escalating dose causes hypotension	Escalating dose causes bradycardia

CHAPTER 4

Hypnotics and Sedatives

DEFINITIONS

- **Sedatives:** Agents which depress central nervous system (CNS) activity producing a calming effect or drowsiness.
- **Hypnotics:** Agents which facilitate the onset and maintenance of sleep.

HISTORY

- Alcoholic beverages, laudanum and some herbs were used to induce sleep.
- Bromide was the first agent to be used as sedative hypnotic in the middle of the nineteenth century.
- Other agents like chloral hydrate, paraldehyde, sulfonal and urethane were also used.
- Phenobarbital was introduced in 1912.
- Chlordiazepoxide synthesized by Sternbach, actions explained by Randall, was introduced for use in 1961. Thus began the era of benzodiazepines.
All agents with sedative hypnotic effects may be broadly classified as benzodiazepines, barbiturates, nonbenzodiazepines or Z-compounds. Sedation may be an adverse effect of the other agents like antihistaminics, antipsychotics, or other central nervous system (CNS) depressants like alcohol.

CLASSIFICATION

Benzodiazepines

- Ultrashort acting (t½ <½ hr), e.g. Midazolam.
- Short acting (t½ <6 hr), e.g. Triazolam.
- Intermediate-acting (t½:6–24 hr), e.g. Temazepam.
- Longacting (t½: >24 hr), e.g. Diazepam.

Barbiturates

- *Ultrashort-acting*: Thiopentone sodium and methohexitone.

- *Shortacting*: Pentobarbitone and butobarbitone.
- *Long-acting*: Phenobarbitone.

Newer Nonbenzodiazepines or Z-compounds
Zolpidem, zaleplon and zopiclone.

Melatonin Congener
Ramelteon.

Others
Buspirone, chloral hydrate and paraldehyde.

MECHANISM OF ACTION

The $GABA_A$-BZD-Cl^- channel receptor is composed of five subunits of α, β, γ and any of δ, ε, θ, or Π subunits. There are multiple subtypes of the benzodiazepine receptor, of which $2\alpha_1$, $2\beta_2$, γ_2 pentamer is most common.

Benzodiazepines
Act selectively on benzodiazepine receptor, an integral part of $GABA_A$ receptor—chloride channel complex; binding site between two α_1 and γ_2 subunits interphase enhances presynaptic and postsynaptic inhibition by:
- Enhancing response to GABA.
- Facilitating opening of GABA-activated chloride channels.

Barbiturates
Act on α or β subunit of $GABA_A$ receptors in central nervous system (CNS), at sites different from that of benzodiazepines and increase the duration of opening of the chloride channels.

Nonbenzodiazepines
Act selectively on GABA receptor isoforms containing α_1 subunits and exert more selective action. As α_2 and α_3 subunits of $GABA_A$ receptor are associated with anxiolytic and muscle relaxant activity, these drugs are devoid of these effects.

Others
Alcohol, intravenous anesthetic agents like propofol, etomidate, thiopentone act on β_2, β_3 subunits of the $GABA_A$ receptor.

Antagonists bicuculline blocks GABA binding while flumazenil is a specific competitive antagonist at the benzodiazepine-binding site.

BENZODIAZEPINES

Pharmacokinetics
- All are absorbed orally.
- Have huge lipid-water distribution coefficient in nonionized form.

- Rate of oral absorption differ according to lipophilicity; most barbiturates and newer hypnotics are absorbed rapidly into the blood.
- Extensive distribution crosses BBB, placental barrier and secreted in milk.
- Plasma protein binding varies markedly (e.g. 99% for diazepam while 10% for flurazepam).
- Metabolized in the liver, many produce active metabolites, e.g. flurazepam, diazepam, chlordiazepoxide, alprazolam.
- Ultrarapid elimination seen with triazolam and midazolam.
- Half-life 2–40 hours; long half-life as with diazepam, flurazepam, lorazepam and clonazepam.
- Metabolites are excreted in urine as glucuronide conjugates.

Actions

Anxiolysis and muscle relaxation produced by benzodiazepines are mediated through γ subunit, whereas its anticonvulsant action is mediated through α_1-subunit of $GABA_A$ receptor. The site of action of muscle relaxation is at spinal cord level and requires higher doses than the doses required for other actions.

- Reduction of anxiety and aggression.
- Sedation and induction of sleep.
- Reduction of muscle tone and coordination.
- Anticonvulsant effect.
- Anterograde amnesia.
- Do not have antidepressant effect; poor analgesia.
- May increase irritability and aggression in some individuals.
- Benzodiazepine withdrawal symptoms more commonly seen with short-acting compounds.

Hypnosis

- Hasten onset of sleep.
- Increase total duration of sleep.
- Proportion of rapid eye movement (REM) sleep is reduced.
- Duration of stage 2 non-rapid eye movement (NREM) is increased.
- Duration of stage 4 non-rapid eye movement (NREM) sleep is decreased.
- Growth hormone secretion remains unaffected.
  Abrupt cessation of drug may result in rebound in REM sleep; tolerance develops if drug is used for > 4–6 weeks.

Sedation

Sedation is a function of GABA receptors containing α_1 subunit.
- Calming effect at relatively low doses.
- Depressant effects on psychomotor and cognitive functions.
- Euphoria.
- Impaired judgement, loss of self-control.
- Dose-dependent anterograde amnesia.

Other Actions

- *Anesthesia*: IV anesthesia, induction of anesthesia; diazepam, midazolam, lorazepam.
- *Muscle relaxation*: Inhibitory effect on polysynaptic reflexes and internuncial neurons; meprobamate and diazepam.
- *Anticonvulsant*: Clonazepam, diazepam, lorazepam and nitrazepam.
- *Respiratory and cardiovascular system*: Dose related depression of medullary respiratory center and or vasomotor center causing respiratory depression or circulatory collapse.
- Anxiolytic and anterograde amnesia are the most desired effects; also utilized in premedication.

Adverse Effects

- Dizziness, headache, vertigo and ataxia.
- Amnesia, delayed reaction time and impaired psychomotor skills.
- Weakness, blurring of vision, dry mouth and urinary incontinence.
- Paradoxical actions, e.g. Irritation, anger.
- Tolerance and cross-tolerance.

Drug Interactions

- Synergistic with alcohol and other central nervous system (CNS) depressants.
- CYP/3A4 inhibitors, e.g. ketoconazole, erythromycin, cimetidine, INH, oral contraceptive pills (OCP) retard benzodiazepine metabolism.

Uses

- *Anxiety states*: Generalized anxiety disorders, panic disorders and agoraphobia.
- *Sleep disorders*: Newer nonbenzodiazepine hypnotics are better.
- *Seizure disorders*: Diazepam, clonazepam.
- *IV anesthesia*: Midazolam, diazepam.
  Preanesthetic medication
  In short surgical procedures, e.g. bronchoscopy and diagnostic procedures
  To control symptoms of ethanol or other hypnotic sedative withdrawal.

BARBITURATES

Classification

- *Long-acting*: Phenobarbitone.
- *Short-acting*: Butobarbitone and pentobarbitone.
- *Ultrashort-acting*: Thiopentone and methohexitone.
- Barbiturates are substituted derivatives of barbituric acid; general CNS depressants; cause dose-dependent—anxiolysis, amnesia, hypnosis, anesthesia, coma and respiratory depression.

Pharmacokinetics

- Half-life 4–60 hours.
- Orally absorbed and widely distributed.
- Onset of action dependent on lipid solubility.
- Plasma protein binding varies; cross-placenta.
- Termination of action depends on redistribution effect, metabolism and excretion.
- Barbiturates with low-lipid solubility are excreted unchanged in urine.
- Barbiturates induce hepatic microsomal enzymes.

Uses

- *Epilepsy*: Phenobarbitone.
- *Anesthesia*: Thiopentone.
- *Hypnotic*: Secobarbital.
- *Congenital nonhemolytic jaundice and kernicterus*: Phenobarbitone.

Adverse Effects

Hangover, tolerance, dependence, idiosyncrasy, precipitation of porphyria in susceptible patients.

NEWER HYPNOTICS

Special Features

- Rapid onset of hypnosis.
- Minimum incidence of hangover, amnesic or psychomotor depressant action.
- Sleep pattern is minimally affected; withdrawal effect is not seen on discontinuation.
- Anticonvulsant, antianxiety or muscle relaxation effects are not evident especially with zolpidem.
- Short duration of effect.
- No tolerance or dependence noted.

Drugs

Eszopiclone, zaleplon and zolpidem.

Uses

Insomnia especially with prolonged sleep latency.

Ramelteon

- Melatonin receptor agonist.
- Activates MT_1 and MT_2 melatonin receptors in suprachiasmatic nuclei of central nervous system (CNS).

Hypnotics and Sedatives 51

- Rapid onset of sleep; minimal rebound insomnia or withdrawal symptoms.
- Orally active; active metabolite.
- *Adverse effects*: Dizziness, fatigue, decreases testosterone, increases prolactin.
- Used for sleep onset insomnia.

Flumazenil

- Benzodiazepine analogue with minimum intrinsic activity.
- Acts on benzodiazepine receptor and reverses the activity of benzodiazepines and zolpidem, zaleplon and zopiclone, no other sedative—hypnotics.
- Used IV; short half-life; oral bioavailability 16%.
- After IV injection-action starts within seconds and lasts for 1-2 hours.
- Reverses the hypnogenic, psychomotor, cognitive and EEG effects.
- Used in benzodiazepine overdose—0.2 mg/min IV.

BUSPIRONE

- Partial agonist at $5HT_{1A}$ receptors, may have activity against D_2 receptors as well.
- Slow onset of action; 1-2 weeks; no withdrawal symptoms or abuse liability.
- Anxiolytic action with minimum psychomotor impairment.
- No additive effect when given along with central nervous system (CNS) depressant drugs.
- *Orally active*: Active metabolite; short ½ life.
- *Adverse effects*: Tachycardia, paresthesia and GI distress.

COMPARATIVE STUDY OF COMMONLY USED DRUGS

Barbiturates

Drug	Indications	Dose	Comments
Phenobarbitone	Generalized tonic-clonic seizure, partial seizure; sedative hypnotic	15–20 mg 2–3 times/day	Prolonged duration of action; induce hepatic microsomal enzymes
Thiopentone 25 mg/mL in solution + 1.5 mg/mL Na_2CO_3	Ultrashort-acting intravenous anesthetic	Induction dose 2.5% solution 3–5 mg/kg	Duration 5–8 min, Highly alkaline, pH 10–11
Methohexital 10 mg/mL in solution + 1.5 mg/mL Na_2CO_3	Ultrashort-acting intravenous anesthetic	Induction dose 4–7 mg/kg	Duration of induction 4–7 min; pH 10–11

Benzodiazepines

Drug	Indications	Dose	Comments
Diazepam	As hypnotic sedative, anticonvulsant, IV anesthetic	Oral, IM, IV, rectal 0.1–0.2 mg/kg; max 60 mg/day 5–10 mg tab/day; 2.5–5 mg suppository; 0.3–0.5 mg/kg for induction	Several active metabolites, sedation, minimal drug interactions
Lorazepam	As sedative, hypnotic	Oral, IM, IV; 1–2 mg OD/BD	Slower onset, more potent, profound amnesia
Midazolam	As IV anesthetic for induction and maintenance; anti-hallucinatory and anticonvulsant	IV, IM; premedication 0.07–0.08 mg/kg IM; induction 0.15–0.3 mg/kg; infusion 0.02–0.1 mg/kg/hr	Rapid onset of action; duration 6–8 min; liable to abuse, rapid metabolism
Alprazolam	Anxiety disorders	Oral	Intermediate-acting, withdrawal effect, residual effect present
Clonazepam	Seizure disorders, acute mania	Oral	Tolerance may develop
Chlordiazepoxide	Insomnia, anxiety disorders, anesthetic premedication, alcohol withdrawal	Oral, IM, IV 0.3–0.5 mg/kg/day; 10–25 mg tab BD	Long-acting, produce active metabolites
Flurazepam	Insomnia	Oral; 15–30 mg/day	Long-acting
Nitrazepam	Insomnia	Oral; 0 0.5–1 mg/kg/day OD/BD	Long-acting
Temazepam	Insomnia	Oral; 7.5–15 mg/day	Intermediate-acting

Newer Benzodiazepines

Zolpidem	Insomnia	Oral; 5–10 mg at bed time	↓ REM sleep
Zaleplon	Insomnia	Oral; 5–20 mg at bed time	Shortest acting
Eszopiclone	Insomnia	Oral; 1–3 mg at bed time	↑ total sleep time

CHAPTER 5

Skeletal Muscle Relaxants

INTRODUCTION

Drugs that reduce muscle tone by acting peripherally at neuromuscular junction, muscle fiber itself or at the cerebrospinal axis, either to produce muscle paralysis, called neuromuscular blockers or to reduce spasticity in painful muscle spasms, termed spasmolytics. Neuromuscular blockers are generally used with general anesthetic agents to provide muscle relaxation.

CLASSIFICATION

Neuromuscular blockers may be classified broadly into two groups:

Nondepolarizing Muscle Relaxants

These can again be *classified according to duration of action* into:
1. Long-acting—d-tubocurarine, pancuronium, doxacurium, pipecuronium.
2. Intermediate acting—vecuronium, atracurium, cisatracurium, rocuronium.
3. Short acting—mivacurium and gantacurium.

They can also be classified according to chemical structure into:
1. Benzylisoquinolines—atracurium, cis-atracurium, mivacurium, doxacurium, metocurine, d-tubocurarine (cyclic benzylisoquinoline).
2. Aminosteroid—pancuronium, vecuronium and rocuronium.
3. Mixed onium chlorofumarate—gantacurium.

Depolarizing Muscle Relaxants
- Succinylcholine.
- Decamethonium.

FEATURES COMMON TO ALL MUSCLE RELAXANTS

- All are polar quaternary compounds.
- Do not cross blood–brain barrier.
- Poorly lipid-soluble.

Structure Activity Relationship

- Succinylcholine structurally comprises two molecules of ACh-linked together by methyl group; its long slender flexible structure allows it to activate the cholinergic receptor at motor end plate.
- Nondepolarizing muscle relaxants are bulky rigid molecules, containing portions similar to ACh but do not activate the nicotinic cholinergic receptor.
- Pancuronium the bisquarternary aminosteroid is most closely related to ACh and its ACh-like fragments render its high degree of neuromuscular blocking activity.
- Benzylisoquinolinium compounds are more likely to release histamine compared to the aminosteroid compounds due to its content of a tertiary amine.

Actions

1. *Skeletal muscles*: Nondepolarizing agents bind to nicotinic ACh receptors at motor end plate and prevent the binding of acetylcholine (ACh) to the receptors by competitive blockade causing flaccid paralysis.
   Depolarizing muscle relaxants bind to nicotinic ACh receptors and cause persistent depolarization, resulting in initial fasciculation followed by paralysis. In presence of high concentration of depolarizing agent the depolarizing block (phase1 block) may be converted to phase II block which is similar to nondepolarizing block.
   Sequence of block—Smaller muscles of the eyelid, jaw and larynx are paralyzed before the muscles of limbs and trunk. The diaphragm is the last muscle to be paralyzed when respiration totally ceases.
2. *Autonomic ganglia*: Ganglionic blockade is variable with d-tubocurarine having maximum action, producing hypotension and tachycardia, others having minimum effect at clinical doses. Succinylcholine may cause stimulation as observed due to bradycardia (vagal ganglia) or hypertension and tachycardia (sympathetic ganglia).
3. *CNS*: All neuromuscular blockers being quarternary compounds do not cross the BBB and are devoid of any central effects.
4. *Histamine release*: It occurs due to direct action on mast cells. Tubocurarine may cause wheals, bronchospasm, hypotension, increased bronchial and salivary secretions due to histamine release. Succinylcholine, atracurium, mivacurium may cause histamine release. The ammonio steriod group of muscle relaxants have less propensity to release histamine.

PHARMACOKINETICS (TABLE 5.1)

Quarternary ammonium compounds are poorly absorbed through GIT but rapid onset of action occurs when administered IV, absorption is also adequate from after IM administration.

The ammonio steroid compounds are hydrolized of their ester groups in liver, the metabolites too contribute partially to the relaxant activity.

Table 5.1: Comparative properties of commonly used muscle relaxants.

Drug	Onset of action	Duration of action	Excretion	Intubation dose mg/kg	Maintenance dose mg/kg	Infusion rate µg/kg/min
Succinylcholine	1 min	8 min	Plasma cholinesterase	0.5–1	0.04–0.07	—
Tubocurarine	6 min	80 min	Kidney and liver	0.6	0.25–0.5	2–3
Metocurine	4 min	110 min	Kidney	0.4	0.5–1	—
Atracurium	3 min	35 min	Hofmann elimination	0.5	0.08–0.1	5–10
Cis-atracurium	2 min	45 min	Hofmann and renal	0.1–0.4	0.03	1–3
Mivacurium	2 min	15 min	Plasma cholinesterase	0.15–0.25	0.1	9–10
Doxacurium	4 min	120 min	Renal	0.03–0.06	0.005–0.01	—
Pancuronium	3 min	85 min	Renal and hepatic	0.08–0.1	0.01–0.015	1
Vecuronium	2 min	40 min	Renal and hepatic	0.1	0.01–0.015	0.8–1
Rocuronium	1–2 min	35 min	Hepatic	0.6–1.2	0.1–0.2	0.1–0.2
Gantacurium	1 min	10 min	Ester hydrolysis	0.2–0.5	—	—

Vecuronium and **rocuronium** are more rapidly cleared by the liver than **pancuronium**. Atracurium and **cisatracurium** undergo spontaneous degradation or Hofmann elimination and also by plasma esterases, hence can be safely administered in patients with impaired renal function. Succinylcholine is degraded by butyrylcholinesterase synthesized by the liver and found in the plasma. **Mivacurium** is also degraded by plasma cholinesterase. **Gantacurium** is degraded by a two-step chemical reactions, initially addition of cysteine, next slow hydrolysis of ester bond by enzymatic activity.

Clinical Uses

- Muscle relaxation—as an adjuvant to general anesthesia.
- In severe laryngospasm.
- Prior to intubation in intensive therapy unit (ITU).
- During electroshock therapy—to prevent trauma.
- As supportive therapy in severe tetanic spasms.

Adverse Effects

- Prolonged apnea.
- Histamine release and precipitation of bronchospasm.
- Hypotension in hypovolemic patients.
- Hyperkalemia, may induce cardiac dysrhythmia.
- Postoperative muscle pain.

Characteristics of Nondepolarizing Block

- No muscular fasciculation seen.
- Onset of action is slow.
- Muscle can be stimulated by other stimuli like electrical, mechanical even after block.
- In partial paralysis, neuromuscular monitoring shows (Fig. 5.1):
  - Depression of muscle twitch
  - Fade in TOF
  - Post-tetanic facilitation is followed by exhaustion.
- Potentiated by adrenaline, acetylcholine and succinylcholine.
- Mild cooling antagonizes block.
- Cooling below 33°C potentiates block.
- Metabolic acidosis prolongs and intensifies block.
- Potentiated by volatile agents and magnesium.
- Reversed by neostigmine and other anticholinesterases.
- Slow dissociation constant at receptors.
- Repeated tetanic bursts cause their effect to wear off.

Characteristics of Depolarizing Block

- Cause muscular fasciculation.
- Tone of some muscles like ocular muscles increase, decrease in IOT.
- Quick onset of action.
- Muscle cannot be stimulated further, after block.

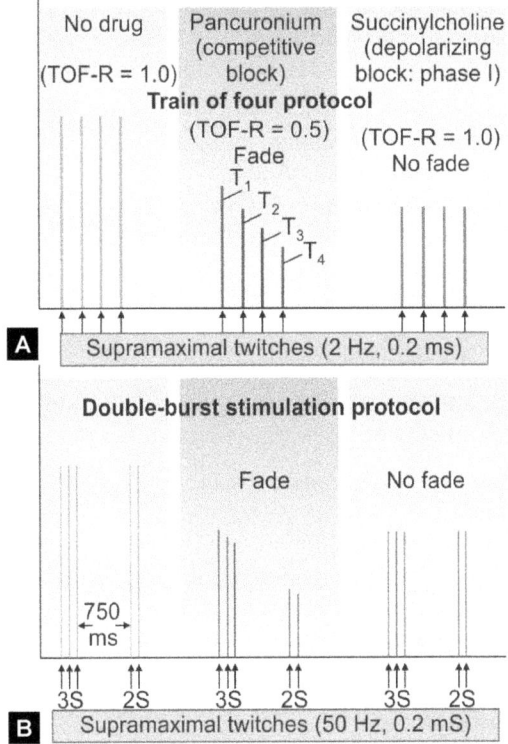

Figures 5.1A and B: Partial paralyzed muscle on neuromuscular monitoring.

- Partial paralyzed muscle on neuromuscular monitoring shows (Fig. 5.1):
  - Depression of twitch
  - No fade
  - No post-tetanic facilitation
- Potentiated by isoflurane, metabolic alkalosis, magnesium.
- Antagonized by metabolic acidosis, nondepolarizing muscle relaxants.
- Not reversed by neostigmine.
- Fast dissociation constant at receptors.
- Repeated stimulation leads to phase II block (which dose of succinylcholine exceeds 3–5 mg/kg IV).
- Phase II block resembles block produced by nondepolarizing muscle relaxants.

Neuromuscular Block Monitoring

Clinical assessment of any residual block at the time of recovery from GA:
- Grip strength.
- Adequate coughing.
- Ability to sustain head lifting for at least 5 seconds.
- Adequate vital capacity of 10 mL/kg body weight.
- Ability to produce negative inspiratory effort of at least 20 cm H_2O against an obstructed airway.
- Absence of tracheal tug or paradoxical breathing.

Nerve stimulators can be used to assess the depth of block or adequate reversal from neuromuscular blockade.

Charcteristics
- Duration of impulse—0.1–0.3 ms.
- Supramaximal current 50–60 mA.
- Frequencies used—0.1 Hz, 2 Hz, 50 Hz.
- Types—single twitch, train of four, tetanic stimulus, post-tetanic count, double burst stimulus.

Nerves Stimulated
- Ulnar, posttibial, facial, common peroneal nerves.
- Contraction of muscles can be assessed visually, palpated or measured with pressure transducer.

Conditions where nerve stimulators are used:
- Prolonged apnea.
- Neostigmine resistant cases.
- Patients with liver or kidney dysfunction.
- Myasthenia gravis or myasthenic syndrome.
- If suxamethonium infusion is used.

Conditions which prolong neuromuscular blockade:
- Respiratory acidosis.
- Metabolic alkalosis.
- Hypothermia.
- Hypokalemia.
- Hypermagnesemia.
- Coadministration of
    - Antibiotics like streptomycin, neomycin
    - LA like cocaine, procaine and lidocaine
    - Corticosteroids.
- Deranged liver or kidney function.

Conditions which cause resistance to neuromuscular blockade:
- Antiepileptic drugs and chronic phenytoin therapy.
- Patients with burns due to hyperkalemia.

Succinylcholine Apnea

Prolonged apnea following succinylcholine administration was first reported in 1952. The most common causes are:
- Atypical serum cholinesterase (inherited) as,
    - Mendelian recessive homozygous, 1 in 3000 population who have 1–2-hour apnea during which phase II block develops.
    - Fluoride resistant homozygous have 1 hour apnea with phase II block. In both cases heterozygotes are minimally affected with apnea of maximum 10 minutes duration.
    - Silent gene.

- Low serum cholinesterase (acquired)
  - In these cases about 25 units of cholinesterase is present and apnea occurs for about 25-30 minutes. The causes are:
  - Liver disease and hypoproteinemia
  - Starvation and malnutrition
  - Carcinomatosis
  - Pregnancy and newborn
  - Hyperpyrexia
  - Cardiac failure and uremia
  - Asthma
  - Myxedema
  - Drugs, e.g. etomidate, propanidid, ester LA, methotrexate, MAO-inhibitors, esmolol.
- Plasma cholinesterase antagonism—use of neostigmine.
- Overdose of succinylcholine may result in formation of intermediate product, succinylmonocholine which has 5-20% of activity of succinylcholine or due to phase II block.
- Other associated causes may be responsible, e.g.
  - Cerebral depression, hypocapnea, hypercapnea, metabolic acidosis, depression of lung stretch receptors or reflex laryngeal apnea.

Management

- Intermittent positive pressure ventilation (IPPV) and sedation to be maintained till block wears off.
- Blood sampling for plasma cholinesterase analysis.
- Fresh frozen plasma (contains about 36-40 units/mL).
- Blood transfusion (contains about 30 units/mL).
- Other causes of apnea if present, treated according to cause.
  - Plasma cholinesterase level can be assessed by dibucaine number which is normally 77-83. Homozygotes with deficiency have dibucaine number of less than 30, while heterozygotes have dibucaine number of 45-68.

Postsuccinylcholine Muscle Pain

- Occurs commonly in about 50% of patients exposed to the drug.
- Muscles of shoulder girdle, neck and thorax are mainly involved.
- Pain may mimick viral myositis and may linger till 3-4th postoperative day.
- Incidence greater in muscular adults with repeated dosing. Exact cause not known; does not correlate to the extent of fasciculation.

Prevention of Pain

- Precurarization with about 10% of normal dose of nondepolarizing muscle relaxant, 2-3 minutes before induction of anesthesia.
- A small dose, 0.1 mg/kg body weight of succinylcholine before induction followed by the rest of the dose after 1 minute.

- Diazepam 0.15 mg/kg body weight, IV before induction.
- Dantrolene 2 hours preoperatively.

Adverse Effects of Succinylcholine
- Hyperkalemia.
- Myalgia.
- Myoglobinuria.
- Increased intragastric pressure.
- Increased intraocular pressure.
- Cardiac arrhythmia
    - Sinus bradycardia
    - Junctional rhythm
    - Sinus arrest.

CHAPTER 6

Drugs Used in Reversal of Neuromuscular Block

The action of acetylcholine at the neuromuscular junction is prevented by neuromuscular blocking agents. The acetylcholine released is hydrolyzed by acetylcholinesterase present at the synapses. Drugs which inhibit acetylcholinesterase, is capable of reversing the neuromuscular blockade by increasing acetylcholine concentration at the synaptic cleft.

HISTORY

The first anticholinesterase to be used is physostigmine, also called Eserine, an alkaloid derived from seeds of calabar beans, or physostigma venenosum, is a reversible type of cholinesterase inhibitor. A new class of irreversible cholinesterase inhibitors came into use during World War II and were used as pesticides or as chemical warfare agents.

CLASSIFICATION

1. Noncovalent reversible anticholinesterase, e.g. edrophonium, tacrine, donepezil and propidium.
2. Carbamylating anticholinesterase, e.g. physostigmine, neostigmine and pyridostigmine.
3. Organophosphate anticholinesterase, e.g. DFP, ecothiophate, malathion.

MECHANISM OF ACTION

- Both reversible carbamylating as well as irreversible organophosphates bind covalently to the active center, serine of the acetylcholinesterase enzyme just as acetylcholine.
- Noncovalent reversible acetylcholinesterase inhibitors bind to the choline subsite of the enzyme.
  The acetylcholinesterase enzyme is thus sequestrated and is unable to hydrolyze acetylcholine. Reactivation of noncovalent-binding anticholinesterases, e.g. edrophonium occurrs in <10 minutes by diffusion

and not by hydrolysis, thus duration is brief. Half-life of reactivation of carbamylated enzyme is about 30 minutes while that of phosphorylated enzyme is in days.

The normal duration of action of acetylcholine at the motor end plate is 200 μsec, shorter than the refractory period of the muscle. Thus, the nerve impulse produces a single wave of depolarization on the muscle fiber. When acetylcholinesterase is inhibited, accumulated acetylcholine diffuses laterally and interacts with multiple receptors, successive stimulation of which results in production of end plate potential and depolarization, thereby antidromic firing of motor neuron.

The commonly used drug, neostigmine is capable of reversing the blockade of nondepolarzing muscle relaxants but not depolarizing agents, the action of which may rather be enhanced by neostigmine.

Comparison of commonly used anticholinesterases is listed in Table 6.1.

Other Actions

- Increased secretion of bronchial, salivary, lacrimal, gastric, pancreatic and sweat glands.
- Increased contraction of smooth muscles of bronchioles, gastrointestinal tract (GIT) and ureters.
- *Action on cardiovascular system (CVS)*: Bradycardia, decreased cardiac output, high doses may cause hypotension.
- *Action on ganglia*: Initial excitation followed by blockade.
- *Action on central nervous system (CNS)*: Lipophilic anticholinesterases enter the brain to increase alertness and cognition, higher doses may produce excitement and convulsion, followed by coma.
- *Action on eye*: Miosis, decreased IOT, conjunctival hyperemia.

PHARMACOKINETICS

- Physostigmine is highly lipid soluble and is absorbed from GIT, parenteral sites, crosses blood-brain barrier (BBB), cornea; hence used in treatment of atropine poisoning.
- Neostigmine and pyridostigmine are quarternary ammonium compounds and are not lipid soluble. They are poorly absorbed from GIT, donot cross BBB or cornea. They are partially hydrolyzed by plasma cholinesterases and partially excreted unchanged in urine.
- Organophosphates are lipid soluble, absorbed from all sites, cross BBB, mucous membrane, skin and cornea. They are hydrolyzed or oxidized, little is excreted unchanged in urine. Of the organophosphates ecothiophate is highly polar, do not cross BBB, and is less distributed in the body.

Uses

- As miotic.
- In treatment of myasthenia gravis.
- In treatment of paralytic ileus.
- In reversal of neuromuscular block by nondepolarizing muscle relaxants.
- As prophylactic treatment in cobra bite.

Table 6.1: Comparison of commonly used anticholinesterases.

Drug; (Generic and trade name)	Dosage form	Duration of action	Dose and mode of use	Use
Edrophonium Inj tensilon	10 mg/mL ampoule	10–30 min	2–10 mg IV	Diagnostic test
Physostigmine	Oral tablet, injection in ampoule, eyedrop	4–6 hr	0.5–1 mg oral or parenteral	Glaucoma, atropine poisoning
Neostigmine Inj Prostigmin Tilstigmin, Myostigmin	0.5 mg/mL in 1 mL and 5 mL ampoule	3–4 hr	0.5–2.5 mg IM/IV	Myasthenia gravis, reversal of neuromuscular blockade
Pyridostigmine distinon, myestin, mestinon	60 mg tablet	6–8 hr	60–180 mg tab TDS	Myasthenia gravis, paralytic ileus

Sugamadex

It is a unique neuromuscular reversal drug; a novel cyclodextrin and is the first new class of selective relaxant binding agents, which is capable of reversal of neuromuscular block produced by nondepolarizing muscle relaxants rocuronium and vecuronium. It can act at any stage of moderate-to-deep neuromuscular blockade; the synthetic cyclodextrin molecule acts by encapsulation of rocuronium or vecuronium molecule. The drug does not bind to plasma protein or RBC, does not produce any metabolite and is excreted unchanged mainly in the urine. The minimum effective reversal dose of sugamadex is 2 mg/kg IV and given as single bolus dose within 10 sec.

Myasthenia Gravis

- Chronic autoimmune disorder where there is decreased functional ACh receptors at the neuromuscular junction due to destruction by circulating antibodies.
- Hallmark of the disease is muscle weakness and easy fatiguibility of voluntary muscles on repetitive use with partial recovery on rest.
- Ptosis, diplopia, dysphagia are the initial symptoms, and there is increased sensitivity to non depolarizing muscle relaxants.
- Prevalence is 1 in 7500; women of 20–30 years are most affected.
- Classification is done, based on the skeletal muscles involved and the severity of symptoms.
  - *Type I*: Limited to extraocular muscles, usually nonprogressive.
  - *Type IIa*: Slowly progressive with mild skeletal muscle weakness, response to anticholinesterase drugs and corticosteroids is good.

- *Type IIb*: Rapidly progressive severe form of skeletal muscle weakness, response to drug therapy is not good. Respiratory muscles too may be involved.
- *Type III*: Acute onset and rapid progression. Deterioration of skeletal muscle strength in 6 months; high mortality.
- *Type IV*: Severe form of skeletal muscle weakness that results from progression of type I or type II myasthenia.
- *Other signs and symptoms*: Associated dysphagia, dysarthria, salivation, asymmetric arm, leg or trunk muscle weakness. Myocarditis with AF, heart block or cardiomyopathy can occur. Infection, electrolyte imbalance, emotional stress, pregnancy, antibiotics, e.g. aminoglycosides, increase muscle weakness.
- *Treatment*: Anticholinesterase drugs are first line of therapy. Thymectomy, short-term immunotherapy, immunosuppression, plasmapheresis and immunoglobulin administration are the other modalities of treatment.

Preoperative Preparation

- Optimizing muscle strength, including respiratory function; If VC < 2L, plasmapheresis is to be done before surgery.
- Immunosuppressive therapy should preferably be avoided due to increased risk of perioperative infection; it is only indicated if anticholinesterase drug therapy is inadequate. Corticosteroids, azathioprine, cyclosporine are used.

Intraoperative Specificities

- Induction by short-acting IV anesthetic.
- Tracheal intubation often is done without neuromuscular blocking agents.
- Volatile anesthetic agent is to be used for maintenance of anesthesia, with/without nitrous oxide.
- Nondepolarizing muscle relaxants, if used, should be less than 1/2-2/3rd of normal dose.
- Recovery from anesthesia should be monitored by peripheral nerve stimulator. Extubation should only be done after confirmation of adequate skeletal muscle strength and proper respiratory function.

Postoperative Care

- Ventilatory support is often necessary.
- Neuraxial analgesia decreases postoperative pain.
- Pyridostigmine therapy is to be continued.

CHAPTER 7

Anticholinergic Drugs Used in Anesthesia

INTRODUCTION

1. Natural alkaloids—atropine and hyoscine
2. Semisynthetic derivatives—atropine methonitrate, hyoscine butylbromide, ipratropium bromide, tiotropium bromide. These agents show selectivity for muscarinic receptor subtypes, differing in duration of action from parent compounds (Table 7.1).

ACTIONS OF PROTOTYPE DRUG ATROPINE

- *Action on central nervous system (CNS)*: Mild stimulation of medullary vagal nuclei and higher cerebral centers in therapeutic doses. In toxic doses produce excitation, irritability, restlessness, disorientation and hallucination.
  Hyoscine in contrast, at therapeutic doses cause drowsiness, amnesia, fatigue, dreamless sleep and prevents motion sickness by depressing vestibular excitation.
- *Action on cardiovascular system (CVS)*: Predominant action is tachycardia due to M_2 blockade on SA node. Refractory period of AV node is decreased; PR interval is shortened. BP is not affected. Blocks vasodepressor action of cholinergic agents. Resting heart rate is

Table 7.1: Differences between natural alkaloids atropine and hyoscine.

Characteristics	Atropine	Hyoscine
Chief source (natural)	Atropa belladona	Hyoscyamus niger
Constituent	Tropine + tropic acid	Scopine + tropic acid
Predominant sites of anticholinergic action	Heart, bronchial muscle and intestine	Secretory glands and eye
Duration of action	Long	Short
CNS	Excitatory	Depressant

increased by 35–40 beats/min. In toxic doses cause cutaneous vasodilation, specially in the 'blush area', called the 'atropine flush'.
- *Respiratory tract*: Inhibit bronchial secretion of mouth, nose, pharynx, decrease mucus secretion as well as mucociliary clearance. Decreases airway resistance specially in chronic obstructive pulmonary disease (COPD) and asthma patients.
- *Action on smooth muscles*: Relaxes smooth muscles of ureter, urinary bladder, bronchial muscles; relaxation of biliary tract is less marked and effect on uterus is minimal.
- *Action on gastrointestinal tract (GI tract)*: Relaxation of smooth muscles and decreased secretions including gastric acid. Decreases acid, pepsin and mucin of gastric acid, volume of which is also decreased. Relaxation leads to antispasmodic action but increased sphincteric tone and decreased GI secretion leads to constipation. Mild antispasmodic action on gallbladder and bile ducts.
- *Action on urinary bladder*: Relaxation of detrussor muscles but increase in sphincteric tone may lead to urinary retention specially in elderly.
- *Action on sweat glands and temperature*: Inhibit the action of sweat glands innervated by sympathetic cholinergic fibers. Decreased sweating leads to increase in body temperature.
- *Action on eye*: Topical instillation causes mydriasis, cycloplegia and abolition of light reflex. Photophobia, blurring of vision may result, intraocular tension (IOT) is increased. Mild local anesthetic action on cornea.

PHARMACOKINETICS (TABLE 7.2)

Absorbed from GI tract, on topical instillation, can penetrate cornea. 50% is metabolized in liver, rest is excreted unchanged in urine. Plasma half-life 3–4 hours.

Uses
- Preanesthetic medication.
- Bradyarrhythmias and partial heart block.
- Cardiac arrest.

Adverse Effects
- Dry mouth and difficulty in deglutition.
- Dry flushed skin.
- Difficulty in micturition and decreased bowel movements.
- Dilated pupils and photophobia.

Contraindications
- Narrow angle glaucoma.
- Elderly males with benign hypertrophy of prostate.
- Presence of fever.

Table 7.2: Comparison of commonly used anticholinergic drugs.

Drug; (Generic and trade name)	Dose	Dosage form	Indications	Comments
Atropine; atropine sulfate	0.6–2 mg IM/IV or 10 µg/kg	0.6 mg/mL inj, 1% eye drop, 5% eye ointment	Cardiac arrest, bradyarrhythmias, to counteract cholinergic activity, pre-anesthetic medication prior to decurarization, to correct brady-arrhythmias	Commonly used, CNS actions negligible
Hyoscine; Hyoscine butylbromide	0.3–0.5 mg oral, IM, transdermal	Inj, oral tablet, transdermal patch	Motion sickness, preanesthetic medication	Central depressant action
Glycopyrrolate; Pyrolate, Glyco-P	5–10 µg/kg; 0.1–0.3 mg IM	0.2 mg/mL in 1 mL amp, 1 mg in 5 mL vial	Pre anesthetic medication	Potent, rapid onset of action, no central effects

- Coadministration of drugs like antihistaminics, tricyclic antidepressants (TCA), monoamine oxidase (MAO) inhibitors.

PREANESTHETIC MEDICATIONS

Drugs administered prior to anesthesia in order to:
- Relieve anxiety and apprehension.
- Cause sedation and amnesia.
- Counteract the adverse effects of anesthetic agents, e.g. bradycardia and increased secretions.
- Potentiate analgesia and anesthesia during surgery.
- To decrease the incidence of perioperative nausea and vomiting.
- To decrease the volume of gastric acid secretion and prevent complications like aspiration pneumonia.

The drugs commonly used are:
- Sedatives and anxiolytics, e.g. midazolam, pethidine and fentanyl.
- Anticholinergics, e.g. atropine, hyoscine and glycopyrrolate.
- Antiemetics, e.g. domperidone, ondansetron and granisetron.
- Proton pump inhibitors/H_2 blockers—pantoprazole, lansoprazole, ranitidine and famotidine.
- Analgesics, e.g. pethidine, pentazocine, fentanyl, diclofenac sodium and tramadol.

CHAPTER 8

Nonsteroidal Anti-inflammatory Drugs

INTRODUCTION

- The traditional nonsteroidal anti-inflammatory drugs (NSAIDs) act by inhibiting prostaglandins (PGs); PG-G, PG-H synthesizing enzymes, namely the cyclooxygenases. Cyclooxygenase (COX) exists in two isoforms:
  - COX-1 (constitutive) and COX-2 (inducible), which are responsible for antipyretic, analgesic and anti-inflammatory actions of NSAIDs.
  - Inhibition of COX-1 is responsible for its unwanted GI adverse effects.
- Most NSAIDs inhibit both COX-1 and COX-2.

HISTORY

- Derived from willow bark and leaves; first used by Hippocrates for relief of pain and fever.
- Meadow sweet (Spiraea ulmaria), the plant from which the name aspirin was derived.
- Acetaminophen became popular after 1949.

PATHOPHYSIOLOGY

- Inflammation is a process associated with calor (warmth), rubor (redness), dolor (pain) and tumor (swelling); occurs in response to any obnoxious stimuli, e.g. injury, infection or antibody.
- Various mediators are responsible, e.g. PGs, histamine, bradykinin, leukotrienes, 5-hydroxytryptamine (5HT), platelet-activating factor (PAF).
- PGE_2 and PGI_2 (prostacyclin) are the primary prostanoids that mediate inflammation.
- PGD_2, a major product of mast cells, contributes to inflammation in allergic responses, especially in the lung.
- Activation of endothelial cells plays a key role in 'targeting' circulatory cells to inflammatory sites leading to leukocyte adhesion.
- Cytokines, e.g. IL-6, IL-8, TNF α, β, GM-CSF, etc. are liberated; COX-2 is induced, adhesion molecules, acute-phase proteins further mediate and promote inflammation.

- Glucocorticoids interfere with the synthesis and actions of cytokines such as interleukin-I or tumor necrosis factor α (TNF-α).
- Action of some cytokines is associated with release of prostaglandins (PGs) and thromboxane A_2 (TXA_2); cyclooxygenase (COX) inhibitors appear to block their pyrogenic action.
- Many of the actions of PGs are inhibitory to the immune response and initiate resolution of inflammation.

CLASSIFICATION

A. **Nonselective COX inhibitors:**
- *Salicylates*: Aspirin, salicylate salts and diflunisal.
- *Acetic acid derivatives*: Indomethacin, sulindac and tolmetin.
- *Propionic acid derivatives*: Ibuprofen, fenoprofen, flurbiprofen, ketoprofen, naproxen and oxaprozin.
- *Oxicams*: Piroxicam and meloxicam.
- *Fenamates*: Mefenamic acid and meclofenamic acid.
- *Arylacetic acid derivatves*: Diclofenac and aceclofenac.
- *Pyrazolone derivatives*: Phenylbutazone and oxyphenbutazone.
- *Pyrrolopyrole*: Ketorolac.

B. **Preferential COX-2 inhibitors**: Nimesulide, nabumetone and meloxicam.

C. **Selective COX-2 inhibitors**: Celecoxib, rofecoxib, etoricoxib, parecoxib.

D. **NSAIDs with minimum anti-inflammatory activity**: Paracetamol, metamizol and nefopam.

MECHANISM OF ACTION

Action of NSAIDs is by inhibition of prostaglandin (PG) synthesis, irreversibly by aspirin and reversibly by others. COX exists in two isoforms—COX-1, COX-2. COX-1 is constitutive, present in almost all tissues especially lung and spleen, while COX-2 is inducible, induced by inflammatory cytokines, interleukin, TNF or other pathological stimuli. COX-2 is constitutive in brain and kidney. Inhibition of cyclooxygenase leads to inhibition of PGs, PGE_2, $PGF_2α$, PGI_2, TXA_2 resulting in some beneficial effects like analgesia, antipyresis, anti-inflammatory actions while some toxicities like peptic ulceration, retention of salt and water or enhanced leukotrienes synthesis resulting in precipitation of asthma.

Actions

- *Analgesia*: PGs produced due to trauma or inflammation increase pain sensitivity to bradykinin, TNF-α, interleukins and other analgesics. NSAIDs reduce pain by inhibiting the COXs responsible for liberating PGs.
- *Antipyresis*: Hyperthermia induced by PGE_2 in hypothalamus due to pyrogens, ILs, TNF-α, etc. is inhibited by NSAIDs and temperature is reset to normal.

- *Anti-inflammatory*: Inhibition of PG synthesis at the site of injury reduces inflammation.
- *Action in GIT*: NSAIDs inhibit the gastro-protective action of PGs on gastric mucosa. Deficiency of PGs leads to increased acid secretion, decreased mucus and bicarbonate production resulting in mucosal erosion or ulceration with/without bleeding. Paracetamol and COX-2 inhibitors have minimum effect. PGE analogue, misoprostol is used to treat NSAIDs-induced ulcer.
- *Action in kidney*: COX-1 inhibition by NSAID causes decreased renal blood flow, decreased GFR leading to renal insufficiency; increased Na^+ and water retention may lead to edema. Inhibition of PG synthesis in kidney may result in papillary necrosis/analgesic nephropathy.
- *Action on platelets*: NSAIDs inhibit synthesis of both TXA_2 and PGI_2 but action on platelet TXA_2 predominates thereby inhibiting platelet aggregation, increase bleeding time.
- *Action on ductus arteriosus*: Administration of NSAIDs in late pregnancy may cause premature closure of ductus arteriosus by inhibiting PGE_2 and PGI_2 which keep the duct patent during fetal life.
- *Effects on labor*: NSAIDs may delay onset of labor by inhibiting PGs responsible for triggering preterm labor.
- *Anaphylactoid reactions*: Precipitation of asthma, angioneurotic edema, urticaria as a result of inhibition of COX and increased synthesis of LTs via the lipoxygenase pathway.

ASPIRIN

Acetylsalicylic acid converted in the body to salicylic acid.

Mechanism of Action

Acetylate the COX enzymes irreversibly and inhibit PG synthesis.

At higher concentration NSAIDs reduce production of superoxide radicals, decrease proinflammatory cytokines, decrease nitric oxide synthase and induce apoptosis. Inhibition of platelet COX-1 dependent TXA_2 formation is responsible for prevention of platelet aggregation, takes 8–12 days to recover once the therapy is stopped.

Pharmacokinetics of NSAIDs

- Absorbed rapidly followed by oral ingestion.
- Peak plasma level reached in 2–3 hours.
- Food may interfere with bioavailability.
- Some NSAIDs like diclofenac, nabumetone undergo first-pass metabolism.
- High plasma protein binding.
- Well distributed; some attain high concentration in synovial fluid (Half the plasma concentration → Ibuprofen, naproxen, piroxicam; similar to plasma concentration → Indomethacin; higher than plasma concentration → Tolmetin).

- Most NSAIDs reach CNS in sufficient concentration.
- COX-2 inhibitors attain high concentration at sites of inflammation.
- Hepatic biotransformation followed by renal excretion occurs.
- Some have active metabolites like fenbufen, nabumetone, meclofenamic acid.
- Pharmacokinetics of aspirin is altered due to age variation and disease conditions.

Uses
- Musculoskeletal disorders as anti-inflammatory agent.
- Treatment of ankylosing spondylitis, osteoarthritis, rheumatoid arthritis, gout.
- Bartter syndrome.
- In acute low to moderate degree of pain, e.g. postoperative pain.
- As an alternative to centrally acting analgesics to avoid respiratory depression.
- To counteract flushing during niacin therapy.
- As antipyretic.
- In the closure of PDA.
- As antiplatelet agent in the prevention of stroke and myocardial infarction (MI).
- Systemic mastocytosis.
- Keratolytic action of salicylate utilized in the treatment of warts and corns.

Adverse Effects
- *GI*: Nausea, vomiting, pain abdomen, diarrhea, GI, peptic ulcer and erosion.
- *CNS*: Headache, dizziness, confusion and vertigo.
- *CVS*: MI, stroke and thrombosis.
- *Platelets*: Inhibited activation with increase risk of hemorrhage
- Closure of patent ducts arteriosus (PDA).
- *Renal*: Salt and water retention, hypertension and analgesic nephropathy.
- *Hypersensitivity*: Vasomotor rhinitis, generalized urticaria, bronchial asthma, hypotension and shock.
- *Reye's syndrome*: In children/young adults <20 years; fever, acute encephalopathy, hepatic dysfunction, fatty liver; may be fatal. Seen with aspirin/other salicylates, when administered in viral fever.
- Prolongation of labor and gestation and increase incidence of PPH if used in pregnancy.

Special Adverse Effects of Aspirin
- *Respiration*: Salicylates increase O_2 utilization, increase CO_2 production → stimulation of respiratory center → respiratory rate and depth → respiratory alkalosis.

- *Acid-base and electrolyte balance*: Increased excretion of HCO_3^-, Na^+, K^+ (compensated respiratory alkalosis). High-dose aspirin/NSAIDs cause papillary necrosis and interstitial nephritis.
- *Uricosuric effect*: In high dose, > 5 g/day induce uricosuria.
- *Effects on blood*: Doses > 3-4 g/day can decrease serum iron level; may cause hemolysis in patients with deficiency of Gl-6-PO_4 dehydrogenase.
- *Liver*: Reye's syndrome.
- Large doses may cause hyperglycemia and glycosuria.
- *Ototoxicity*: Tinnitus and hearing impairment may occur due to increased labyrinthine pressure secondary to vasoconstriction of auditory microvasculature; due to direct action of salicylic acid (not due to inhibition of PG).

Therapeutic plasma concentration of aspirin; < 20 μg/mL, for salicylate < 60 μg/mL. For rheumatic diseases, salicylate plasma concentration of 150-300 μg/mL is acceptable. Toxicity appears with plasma concentration > 300 μg/mL. Dose of aspirin as analgesic antipyretic is 324-1000 mg/4-6 hourly.

OTHER SALICYLATES IN USE

- *Diflunisal*: Diflrophenyl derivative of salicylic acid has potent anti-inflammatory action but is devoid of antipyretic action. Used in treatment of painful arthritic conditions as 1 g → 500 mg/8-12 hourly dose.
- *Mesalamine (5-aminosalicylic acid)*: Used in the treatment of inflammatory bowel disease.
- *Olsalazine*: Used in inflammatory bowel disease especially ulcerative colitis.
- *Salicylic acid*: Used for keratolytic action in skin disorders; treatment of corn, wart.
- *Methylsalicylate (oil of wintergreen)*: It used in analgesic ointments for musculoskeletal pain.

ACETAMINOPHEN (PARACETAMOL)

- Active metabolite of phenacetin.
- Analgesic, antipyretic with minimum anti-inflammatory action as it is unable to inhibit COX enzyme at inflammatory sites due to presence of peroxides.
- Well tolerated as analgesic in chronic osteoarthritis due to minimum GI effects.
- COX inhibition in brain is more pronounced compared to other NSAIDs explaining its good antipyretic action.
- Primarily detoxified in liver by glucuronidation but a small part is r-hydroxylated by CYPs to form N-acetyl-p-benzoquinone imine (NAPQI), a harmful metabolite. This NAPQI is attached to sulfhydryl group of glutathione for detoxification. If large doses of acetaminophen is administered, there is accumulation of NAPQI, especially in children

resulting in hepatotoxicity. So, use of higher dose is contraindicated (C/I) in children of 2-11 years; dose of 10 mg/kg body weight is used.
- *Side effect (S/E)*: Rash, fever, allergic manifestations. Hepatotoxicity with high doses.

Acetaminophen Toxicity
- Occurs with intake of > 7.5 g.
- Hepatic dysfunction and depletion of glutathione.
- Renal tubular necrosis.
- Hypoglycemic coma.
- Symptoms like nausea, vomiting, jaundice, tender hepatomegaly, coagulopathy, right subcostal pain, etc. appear within 2-3 days.
- *Treatment*: N- acetylcysteine, in loading dose of 150 mg/kg by infusion in 200 mL of 5% dextrose over 1 hour.

INDOMETHACIN

- Methylated indole derivative.
- Non-selective inhibitor of COX.
- Pronounced anti-inflammatory action, inhibiting polymorphonuclear cell infiltration, decrease mucopolysaccharide synthesis and causing vasoconstriction.
- Good oral bioavailability; peak plasma concentration in 2 hours.
- Undergoes enterohepatic circulation (t½ = 2.5 hours).
- Used for its anti-inflammatory, analgesic and antipyretic action especially in various joint inflammatory disorders.

Uses: Rheumatoid arthritis, Osteoarthritis, Gouty Arthritis, frozen shoulder, ankylosing spondylitis.
- FDA-approved use in closure of PDA in premature infants.

Adverse effects: GI effects like nausea, vomiting, diarrhea, pancreatitis, hepatitis, CNS effects like dizziness, headache, confusion, seizures, psychosis, suicidal tendencies.

Contraindications: Renal failure, hyperbilirubinemia, thrombocytopenia, enterocolitis.

Special precautions: Elderly patients, history of epilepsy, psychiatric disorders, parkinsonism, hemopoietic disorders. Drug interactions with furosemide, thiazides, ACE inhibitors, ARBs.

SULINDAC

- Prodrug, inhibitor of COX; congener of indomethacin but half as potent.
- Produces active metabolite so t½ of 7 hours is prolonged as t½ of active sulfide metabolite is 18 hours.
- Toxicity is lower than indomethacin.

Uses: Acute gout, spondylitis, painful shoulder, tendinitis, bursitis and other painful inflammatory joint disorders.

Side effects: GI effects, rash, pruritus, increase hepatic enzymes.

TOLMETIN

- Bears typical NSAID properties and S/E.
- Efficacy equivalent to moderate doses of aspirin in treatment of osteoarthritis or rheumatoid arthritis.
- Dose: 200–600 mg.

Side effects: GI and CNS effects as indomethacin but less severe.

KETOROLAC

- Acetic acid derivative with potent analgesic and moderate anti-inflammatory activity.
- Administered IM, IV or orally especially in postoperative pain.
- Quick onset of action with short duration.

Other uses: Seasonal allergic conjunctivitis, postoperative ocular inflammation.

Side effect: GI, renal, hypersensitivity and bleeding are main adverse effects.

NABUMETONE

- Prodrug with pronounced anti-inflammatory action.
- Used in rheumatoid arthritis and osteoarthritis.
- Minimum adverse effects.
- Active metabolites (t½ = 24 hours).
- Dose 1000 mg once daily.

DICLOFENAC

- Phenylacetic acid derivative with potent analgesic, anti-inflammatory and antipyretic activity.
- Has COX-2 selective activity and similar to celecoxib.
- Available as potassium or sodium salt.
- Rapid absorption, highly protein bound, extensive first pass metabolism (50%) (t½ = 1–2 hours).
- Higher dose hence is necessary, usual dose 100–200 mg/day.
- Used orally as well as topically in rheumatoid arthritis, osteoarthritis, ankylosing spondylitis, migraine, and dysmenorrhea.

Adverse effects: Mainly GI, modest but reversible elevation of hepatic transaminases. Others are renal, hypersensitivity reactions, CNS effects.

IBUPROFEN

- Most commonly used propionic acid derivative NSAID.
- Nonselective COX-2 inhibitor.
- Rapidly absorbed, highly protein bound, metabolized in liver, excreted in urine.
- Available as tablets, capsules, oral drop suspension; injection available for use in PDA, pain and fever.

Side effect: CNS effects, thrombocytopenia and rashes.

OTHER PROPIONIC ACID DERIVATIVES

Naproxen
About 99% plasma protein bound, t½ is variable, comparatively longer t½ about 14 hours. Metabolites are excreted almost entirely in urine. Adverse effects are similar to other NSAIDs.

Ketoprofen
Potent S-enantiomer in addition to inhibition of COX, it stabilizes lysosomal membranes and has antagonistic action to bradykinin. Mild GI effects are decreased if the drug is taken with food.

Flurbiprofen
In addition to its analgesic anti-inflammatory use, it is indicated in intra-operative miosis as ophthalmic solution.

Oxaprozin
Long half-life about 40–60 hours make once daily administration possible.

Oxicams
- These are enolic acid derivatives with nonselective COX inhibitory action.
- Long half-life of these derivatives allows once daily dosing.
- Lornoxicam, however, has quick onset and short duration of action; (t½ = 3–5 hours).
- Piroxicam has additional anti-inflammtory action by inhibiting neutrophil activation as well as inhibition of proteoglycans and collagenase. However, it has more serious GI and skin manifestations compared with other NSAIDs.
- Meloxicam has significantly less GI adverse effects than piroxicam when used at minimum dose.

COX-2 SELECTIVE NSAIDs

- Diaryl heterocyclic cyclooxygenase inhibitors.
- Celecoxib first COX-2 selective NSAIDs to be used.
- Etoricoxib, rofecoxib, valdecoxib, parecoxib, lumiracoxib are the other COX-2 selective agents that were available; but most are banned.
- Discovered in 1988 by Daniel Simmons.
- *Advantage*: Minimum GI adverse effect especially peptic ulceration.
- *Disadvantage*: Increase incidence of stroke, MI due to COX-2 inhibition in blood vessels resulting in decrease synthesis of PGI_2. High BP → atherosclerotic change.
- As TXA_2 synthesis is not inhibited, platelet aggregation is not prevented, chance of clot formation due to platelet plug → higher risk of MI and stroke.
- These drugs are hence indicated in patients with peptic ulceration or history of peptic perforation or bleeding.

- Should be administered in minimum dose for short period of time.
- These drugs should be avoided in patients with hypertension, ischemic heart disease, history of MI or other cardiovascular events.
- Of the COX-2 inhibitors, celecoxib, etoricoxib, parecoxib are available but rofecoxib and valdecoxib have been withdrawn due to cardiovascular adverse effects.
- Etoricoxib has the highest COX-2 selectivity; t½ 24 hours hence administered once daily.
- *Side effects*: Aphthous ulcers, taste alteration and paresthesia.
- Parecoxib, a prodrug of valdecoxib can be administered parenterally and used for short-term postoperative pain relief.
  NSAIDs used topically as gel, ointment or spray—diclofenac, ibuprofen, flurbiprofen, ketoprofen, naproxen, piroxicam, and nimesulide.

COMPARATIVE STUDY OF SOME COMMONLY USED ANALGESICS

Drug; (Generic and trade name)	Dosage form	Dose	Remarks	Precautions
Aspirin, disprin, ecosprin	75/150/325 mg tablet; inj vial (biospirin)	0.3–0.6 g 6 hourly as analgesic; 75–150 mg/day as antiplatelet	Also used in acute rheumatic fever, PET, PDA, familial colonic polyposis	Peptic ulcer, chickenpox, chronic liver disease, diabetics
Diclofenac voveran, diclonac, diclomax	25/50/75 mg tablet TDS; 25 mg/mL or; 75 mg/mL in 3 mL amp	1–3 mg/kg/day in 2–3 divided doses	Potent, good tissue penetration extended action	Adverse effects are minimum
Paracetamol calpol, crocin, pacimol, pyrigesic	0.5–1 g tablet, 80/170/250 mg suppository	60 mg/kg oral, 15 mg/kg rectal, 5 mg/kg IM 6–8 hourly	Toxicity can occur in neonates and children	Hepatic or renal dysfunction
Indomethacin idicin, indocap	25/50/75 mg capsule or suppository	3 mg/kg/day divided thrice daily	Used in pain of inflammation	Epilepsy, pregnant, children, renal disease
Ketorolac ketanov, ketorol	10 mg tab, 30 mg/mL inj	15–30 mg IM/IV	Action like opioids	Pregnant, premedication
Ibuprofen, ibugesic, brufen	400, 600 mg tablet	10–15 mg/kg 4–6 hourly	Closure of PDA, anti-inflammatory analgesic	Asthmatics
Rofecoxib rofetab, rofiz	25–50 mg/day	25–50 mg/day	Rheumatoid arthritis	Contraindications in children, increase risk of CVD

PATIENT-CONTROLLED ANALGESIA

Patient-controlled analgesia (PCA) can be delivered via various routes—IV, SC, epidural, intrathecal or peripheral nerve catheter. It is advantageous due to minimum time interval between dose administrations, continuous background infusion dosage adjustment can be made instantly. Patient compliance is better. PCA provides more safety, better analgesia, few nocturnal disturbances and rapid recovery.

COMMON ADVERSE EFFECTS OF NSAIDs

- *GI*: Nausea, diarrhea, bleeding peptic ulcer, peptic perforation.
- *Platelets*: Altered platelet aggregation.
- *Renal*: Salt and water retention, edema.
- *CVS*: MI, stroke, thrombosis (Coxibs).
- *CNS*: Headache, dizziness.
- *Hypersensitivity reactions*: Urticaria, angiedema, rash, precipitation of asthma in susceptible patients.

CHAPTER 9

Centrally Acting Analgesics/Opioids

INTRODUCTION

- Opiate → compounds structurally related to opium ('*opos*' → Greek word means juice).
- Natural opiates derived from poppy (somniferum papaver). Natural plant alkaloids are—(i) morphine, (ii) codeine, (iii) thebaine.
- Endogenous opioids are naturally occurring ligands for opioid receptor.
- Endorphin or endogenous opioid peptides, e.g. β endorphin.
- Narcotic is a drug which induces narcosis or sleep (word derived from Greek word '*narkotikos*' meaning stupor).
- Opium contains more than 20 distinct alkaloids.

ENDOGENOUS OPIOID SYSTEM

- The endogenous opioid peptides are derived from a distinct large precursor protein, e.g.
  - Encephalin from preproopiomelanocortin
  - Endorphin from preproenkephalin
  - Dynorphin from preprodynorphin.
- Actions of opioid ligands, both exogenous and endogenous are similar.
- The proopiomelanocortin (POMC) sequence contains a variety of nonopioid peptides, including adrenocorticotropic hormone (ACTH), melanin stimulating hormone, β-lipotropin and adrenocorticotrophic hormone, melanin stimulating hormone all are generated by proteolytic cleavage of proopiomelanocortin (POMC).
- The major opioid peptide derived from further cleavage of β-lipotropin is the potent opioid agonist, β-endorphin.
- The anatomical distribution of proopiomelanocortin (POMC) producing cells is relatively limited in the central nervous system (CNS)
  - Arcuate nucleus of hypothalamus.
  - Nucleus tractus solitarius.

Table 9.1: Comparison of opioid receptor agonists.

Agonists	Receptors		
	μ	δ	κ
1. Etorphine	+++	+++	+++
2. Fentanyl	+++		
3. Levorphanol	+++		
4. Methadone	+++		
5. Morphine	+++		+
6. Hydromorphone	+++		+
7. Sufentanil	+++	+	+
8. Metencephalon and leu-enkephalin	++		+++
9. β-endorphin	+++	+++	
10. Dynorphin A	++		+++

- Proencephalin contains multiple copies of metencephalion and single copy of leu-enkephalin.
- Prodynorphin contains three peptides, dynorphin A, dynorphin B and neoendorphin.
- Recently, a family of peptides named endomorphin namely, endomorphin 1, endomorphin 2, have been identified with selectivity toward μ-opioid receptor.

OPIOID RECEPTORS (TABLE 9.1)

- The three opioid receptors δ, μ, and κ belong to the rhodopsin family of GPCRs and share extensive homologies.
- Their effects on CNS function depend on the density and diverse distribution of receptors in the brain and spinal cord.
- These receptors are expressed in a variety of peripheral sites, e.g. blood vessels, heart, lung, airways, gut, inflammatory and circulating cells.
- The classical opioid receptors has an endogenous ligand, nociceptin/orphanin (FQ:N/OFQ) whose binding sites have been found in CNS—cortical regions, ventral forebrain, hippocampus, brainstem and spinal cord; in peripheral cells like basophils, endothelial cells and macrophages.
- Opioid receptor activation results in following intracellular events:
  - Inhibition of adenylyl cyclase activity.
  - Reduced opening of voltage gated Ca^{2+} channels.
  - Stimulation of K^+ current through several channels.
  - Activation of protein kinase-C (PKC) and phospholipase (PLCB).
- Functional consequences of acute and chronic opiate receptor activation are:

Desensitization.

Tolerance: Sustained administration of an opiate (days to weeks) leads to progressive loss of drug effect; Phenomenon can be manifested at intracellular and at organ level.
- Tolerance is time-dependent; occurring over short-term period.
- Reversible over time
- Tolerance develops in variable rates; For example,
  - Little/no tolerance → pupillary miosis.
  - Moderate tolerance → constipation emesis, analgesia and sedation.
  - Rapid tolerance → euphoria.

Dependence: Dependence represents a state of adaptation manifested by withdrawal symptoms produced by cessation of drug exposure; manifested by agitation, hyperalgesia, hyperthermia, hypertension, diarrhea, papillary dilation, dysphoria, anxiety and depression.

Addiction: Behavioral pattern characterized by compulsive use of a drug and overwhelming involvement with its procurement and use.
- Mechanism of development of tolerance—acute desensitization, receptor internalization, endocytosis and sequestration of receptors.
- Morphine the prototype opioid, is a benzylisoquinoline alkaloid, structural modification of which results in other opioids like codeine, hydrocodone, oxycodone, hydromorphone, etc. More complex alteration of molecular structure of morphine results in mixed agonist-antagonist e.g. nalbuphine or antagonist like naloxone.

General characteristics of opioids:
- Highly soluble weak bases
- Highly protein bound
- Largely ionized at physiologic pH.
- Comparison of commonly used opioids is listed in Table 9.2.

Effects

- *Analgesia*: Analgesia produced by morphine like drugs is associated with drowsiness, changes in mood, mental clouding. Some may experience euphoria. Dull pain is relieved more effectively than sharp intermittent pain. Inflammatory pain often referred to as nociceptive pain. Neuropathic pain responds less well to opioid analgesics.
  - Mechanism
    - Opioid agonists act on GPCRs in brain and spinal cord and modulate neurotransmitter release of glutamate, GABA, acetylcholine, NE, 5HT and substance P.
    - The pain inhibitory neuron is indirectly activated by opioids; altering activity of GABA-ergic interneuron; thereby nociceptive transmission in dorsal horn of spinal cord is further inhibited.
    - Monoamines provide sensory input to higher centers and cause elevation of mood, e.g. NE and 5HT.
    Opiate binding to receptor is highly expressed in the superficial spinal dorsal horn (substantia gelatinosa).

Table 9.2: Comparison of commonly used opioids.

Drug; (Generic and trade name)	Type	Dose	Dosage form	Indications
Morphine; (Morphine sulfate, Morcontin)	Agonist	0.1–0.2 mg/kg SC 3–4 hrly, 2-5 mg IV as premedicant	2–6 mg IV, 10–15 mg IM, 10–50 mg oral; 3–4 hourly	LVF, postoperative pain, cancer pain, pulmonary edema
Codeine	Agonist	0.3 mg/kg/dose as antitussive; 3 mg/kg/dose as analgesic	Cough linctus	Analgesic, cough suppressant, not recommended in children
Pethidine; (Pethidine HCl)	Agonist	50–100 mg IM/SC	100 mg/2 mL vial, 50–100 mg tablet	Intraoperative, postoperative pain and shivering
Tramadol; (Domadol, contramol, tramazac)	Agonist; metabolite of trazodone	50–100 mg 8 hourly	30/100 mg tablet, 50 mg/mL 2 mL vial	Mild to moderate pain, shivering
Pentazocine (Fortwin, Fortagesic)	Agonist-antagonist	0.5–1 mg/kg/day	25 mg tablet, 30 mg/mL amp	Intraoperative, postoperative analgesic
Naloxone; (Narcotan, Nalox)	Pure antagonist	0.2–0.4 mg IV at 2–3 min interval, max 4–10 mg	0.4 mg/mL, 0.04 mg/2 mL	Morphine/opioid overdose, opioid induced respiratory depression
Naltrexone; (Nalima)	Pure antagonist	50 mg/day orally	50 mg tablet	Deaddiction

- Presynaptically opioids block opening of Ca^{+2} channel and post-synaptically enhances opening of K^+ channels leading to hyperpolarization.
- Prevent release of excitatory neurotransmittes from C fibers.
  Direct application of opiates to a peripheral nerve produce a local anesthetic like action at high concentration that is not reversible with naloxone.
  Euphoria, tranquillity and mood altered by opiates is due to the role of mesocorticolimbic dopamine system.
- *Respiration*: Respiratory depression rarely occurs with standard analgesic dose. Opioids should be used with caution in patients with asthma, chronic obstructive lung disease (COPD), cor pulmonale, hypoxia and decreased respiratory drive.

Normal rate and rhythm of respiration is controlled by respiratory center in ventrolateral medula; pO_2 is measured by chemosensors in carotid and aortic bodies and CO_2 is measured by chemosensors in brainstem. Morphine like opioids depress respiration through MOR and DOR receptors with changes in respiratory pattern; opiates depress the chemosensory receptors of brainstem; thus hypoxic stimulation too is depressed. In addition, opioids increase chest wall rigidity and decrease upper airway patency.
- **Factors exacerbating opiate induced respiratory depression:**
    * *Medications*: General anesthetics, tranquilizer, alcohol and sedative hypnotics.
    * *Sleep*: Normal sleep causes decreased sensitivity of medullary center to CO_2; depressant action of morphine acts an additive factor.
    * *Age*: Newborns and elderly are at greater risk of depression.
    * *Disease*: Opiates causes greater depressant action in patients with chronic cardiorespiratory/renal disease.
    * *COPD*: Increased depression of respiration is seen in patients with COPD/sleep apnea.
- *Sedation*: Drowsiness, cognitive impairment, increased incidence of sedation is seen in dementia, encephalopathies, brain tumors and depressant medications.

Maximal respiratory depression occur within 5-10 minutes of IV morphine, 30-90 minutes after IM/SC. Rapid depressant effects occur with lipid-soluble agents.

CODEINE

- *Methyl-morphine*: Converted in the body to morphine.
- 1/10th analgesic as morphine.
- Partial agonist at μ opioid receptor.
- More selective cough suppressant.
- Orally absorbed; t½ life 3-4 hours.
- Constipation occurs.
- Abuse liability is low, no dependence liability.
- Effective only in mild pain, used to suppress cough.

PETHIDINE/MEPERIDINE

- It is a piperidine derivative.
- Meperidine is the first completely synthetic opioid; fentanyl and its congeners like alfentanil, sufentanil are more complex versions of the phenylpiperidine structure.
- Synthesized as atropine substitute, interacts with opioid receptors; actions blocked by naloxone.
- Analgesic $^1/_{10}$th that of morphine, more than codeine.
- Quick onset of action on IM inj; duration 2-3 hours.
- Sedative, euphoriant, respiratory depressant and abuse liability is present.

- Tachycardia and mydriasis.
- Less histamine release.
- Administered orally/IM; active metabolite (norpethidine).
- Completely metabolized in liver and excreted in urine.
- Overdose causes excitatory effects.
- Used as analgesic, as preanesthetic medication.

FENTANYL

- Pethidine congener—highly potent analgesic.
- 80-100 times more potent than morphine.
- Respiratory depression occurs but cardiovascular side effect minimum.
- Does not release histamine.
- Highly lipid-soluble, enters brain and t½ is less than 4 hours.
- Transdermal patch available, can also be given IV; oral, transmucosal, transnasal and transpulmonary routes of drug delivery are also used.
- Used in chronic pain and in anesthesia.

REMIFENTANIL

- Opioid with rapid onset and offset of action.
- Remifentanil undergoes ester hydrolysis by nonspecific plasma and tissue esterases to an inactive metabolite; hence short t½ of about 5 minutes.
- Most common use is in TIVA along with propofol infusion.

METHADONE

- Synthetic opioid with long half-life.
- Blocks both n-methyl d-aspartate (NMDA) receptors and monoamine reuptake transporters; hence used to treat severe pain.
- Superior analgesia at 10-20% of morphine equivalent dose.
- Has analgesic, respiratory depression, constipation, nausea, vomiting, and antitussive actions similar to morphine.
- Administered orally or IM.
- t½ 24-36 hours; highly protein bound (90%).
- Slow persistent action, sedation is less.
- Used as analgesic or to remove opioid-dependence in addicts.
- Abuse liability is low, slow tolerance development, minimum withdrawal symptoms.
- Dose 2.5 10 mg oral/IM.

TRAMADOL

- Centrally acting analgesic.
- Affinity for opioid receptors low; partially antagonized by naloxone.
- Inhibits reuptake of NA, 5HT and activates monoaminergic inhibition of pain at spinal level.
- Metabolite of antipsychotic trazodone.

- Used in mild to moderate pain, chronic pain including cancer pain but not effective in severe pain.
- Well tolerated, minimum hemodynamic changes; minimum abuse liability.

USES OF MORPHINE AND CONGENERS

- As analgesic—traumatic, visceral, ischemic, postoperative, burn and cancer pain. Epidural, intrathecal, transdermal routes of administration may be additionally used.
- Preanesthetic medication.
- Balanced anesthesia.
- Relief of anxiety and apprehension.
- Acute left ventricular failure (LVF)—morphine is analgesic of choice.
- Cough-codeine, dextromethorphan and levopropoxyphene.
- Diarrhea—diphenoxylate and loperamide are used.
- Shivering—pethidine and tramadol are effective.

AGONIST ANTAGONISTS

Pentazocine

- Weak μ antagonistic and marked k agonistic actions; it is a benzomorphan.
- Analgesia primarily spinal; 30 mg equivalent to 10 mg of morphine.
- Sedation, respiratory depression ⅓-½ of morphine.
- Tachycardia and BP rise due to sympathetic stimulation.
- Dysphoria in high dose.
- Tolerance, physical dependence occurs with repeated dose.
- Nausea, vomiting, biliary spasm and constipation less common.
- Effective orally but high first-pass metabolism.
- Irritant, so not given SC.

Butorphanol

- κ receptor, partial agonist, κ analgesic, more potent than pentazocine.
- Analgesia, respiratory depression less than morphine.
- Less dysphoria compared to pentazocine.
- Weak agonist at high dose with some psychomimetic effects.
- May produce physical dependence, abuse potential is low.
- Used as IM/IV in a dose of 1-4 mg in postoperative painful conditions.
- Contraindication (C/I): Cardiac ischemia.

Buprenorphine

- Synthetic thebaine congener.
- Highly lipid soluble.
- Potent analgesic 25 times more potent than morphine.
- Partial agonistic action on μ receptors, antagonistic action on κ receptors.
- Slower onset and longer duration of action.

Nalbuphine

- κ agonist, μ antagonist similar to buprenorphine; used as analgesic.
- Analgesia lasts for 6–8 hours.
- Postural hypotension occurs.
- Constipation less marked.
- Lower incidence of tolerance, physical dependence.
- Withdrawal syndrome resembles that of morphine but is milder.
- High first-pass metabolism makes it orally inactive.
- Sublingual, IM/IV, intrathecal administration.
- Used in long lasting pain.

OPIOID ANTAGONISTS

- Morphine derivatives with bulky substitution at N_{17} position.
- High affinity for μ receptor, lower affinity for other sites, e.g. δ and κ.

Naloxone

- N-allyl—nor-oxymorphone.
- Competitive antagonist at all opioid receptors, more for μ receptor.
- No subjective or autonomic effects produced.
- Inert when given in absence of an agonist.
- In presence of agonist, it completely and dramatically reverses the opioid effects within 1–3 minutes.
- Normalization of respiration, level of consciousness, pupil size, bowel activity and awareness of pain.
- IV 0.4–0.8 mg antagonizes action of morphine but sedation is less completely reversed.
- At 4–10 mg, it antagonizes the agonistic actions of nalorphine, pentazocine, etc. dysphoria and psychomimetic effects are not much antagonized.
- Antagonizes the action of endogenous opioid peptides.
- Partly antagonizes the respiratory depression produced by N_2O, diazepam.
- Inactive orally due to high first-pass metabolism.
- IV action starts in 2–3 minutes.
- Side effect uncommon, rise in BP and pulmonary edema rarely occur.
- Used mainly to treat opioid-induced respiratory depression and to reverse the effect of opioid during labor.

Naltrexone

- Similar to naloxone.
- Longer duration of action (t½ 10 hours.): 1–2 days.
- Chemically related to naloxone, pure antagonist at opioid receptors.
- Orally effective: 50 mg/day orally can be given in addicts.
- No subjective effects, craving subsides.
- S/E—Nausea, headache; high doses can cause hepatotoxicity.

Nalmephine

- Pure opioid antagonist.
- Hepatotoxicity does not occur.
- Higher oral BA.
- Longer duration of action.

Nalorphine

- Closely related structurally to morphine.
- First specific antagonist used.
- Low doses causes antagonistic actions but at high doses analgesic action mimick morphine.
- μ antagonist but κ and δ receptor partial agonistic action.
- May precipitate withdrawal syndrome, hence not used nowadays.

Clinical uses of Opioids

1. As analgesic — pre- and postoperatively.
    - Severe headache, dysmenorrhea.
    - Labor, trauma and burn.
    - MI and renal colic.
    - Terminal disease, e.g. metastatic cancer.
2. In acute LVF.
3. Along with NSAIDs; supplemented first by weak opioids followed by strong opioid analgesic.

DRUG INTERACTION

- Concentration of opioid may be higher when given along with propofol infusion (perhaps due to the hemodynamic changes induced by propofol).
- When coadministered with volatile anesthetics, opioids dramatically reduce the MAC of the volatile anesthetic.
- Synergistic action is seen when opioids are given along with sedatives.

POINTS TO NOTE

- The metabolism of remifentanil is not dependent on hepatic clearance mechanism, nor is its clearance dependent on kidney. It can be used both in hepatic or renal compromised patients, where morphine is rather contraindicated.
- Morphine is more potent and has slower onset of action in women (probably due to cyclic gonadal hormones and psychosocial faction).
- Dosage reduction is necessary in elderly patients (>65 years of age) and it is applicable for all opioids including remifentanil.
- Morphine and pethidine have clinically active metabolites.

CHAPTER 10

Local Anesthetics

INTRODUCTION

A local anesthetic (LA) binds reversibly to a specific receptor within the pore of the Na^+ channels and when in contact with a nerve trunk can cause both sensory and motor paralysis of the area innervated.

HISTORY

- Cocaine was the first local anesthetic, isolated from the leaves of the coca shrub. Coca leaves were chewed for their stimulatory and euphoriant action.
- Carl Koller introduced it into clinical practice as a topical anesthetic in ophthalmological survey.
- Halstead popularized its use in infiltration and conduction block anesthesia.
- Cocaine, ester of benzoic acid came into disuse for its toxicity and addictive liability.

STRUCTURE

- Typical LA contains a hydrophilic and a hydrophobic moiety separated by an intermediate ester or amide linkage.
- The hydrophilic group is either a tertiary or secondary amine and the hydrophobic group is aromatic.
- Hydrophobicity increases the potency and duration of action of the LA. Receptor site affinity of the LA depends on hydrophobicity, so therapeutic index is decreased and chance of toxicity is increased.
- Smaller molecules dissociate faster than larger molecules from the receptor.
- Sensory and motor fibers are equally sensitive; myelinated > nonmyelinated (same diameter), smaller > larger fibers, thinner > thicker, autonomic > somatic.

MECHANISM OF ACTION

Local anesthetics block conduction by preventing permeability of excitable membrane to Na^+. As action of LA starts, threshold for electrical excitability gradually rises. As action potential (AP) declines, conduction slows and eventually stops. Degree of block depends on how the nerve is stimulated and its resting membrane potential.
- Thinner and nonmyelinated fibers are blocked first.
- Sensation of pain disappears first, followed by loss of sensations of temperature, touch, deep pressure and, finally, motor function.
- Autonomic fibers, small unmyelinated C fibers (pain), small myelinated $A\delta$ fibers (pain, temperature) are blocked before larger myelinated $A\gamma$, $A\beta$, $A\alpha$ fibers mediating postural, touch, pressure and motor function. Block occurs in following sequence:
  Pain → Temperature → Touch → Deep pressure.

PHARMACOKINETICS

- They are weak bases.
- Potency depends on increased lipid solubility, increased protein binding and state of increased ionization.
- Ester type of LA, e.g. procaine is hydrolyzed by pseudocholinesterase.
- Amide type of LA, e.g. lignocaine, mepivacaine, bupivacaine and etidocaine undergoes enzymatic degradation in the liver.
- Toxicity is seen more with ester group of LA due to para-aminobenzoic acid moiety.
- S-enantiomer is less toxic than R-enantiomer pharmacodynamically (undesired actions).

Actions

CNS

Restlessness, tremor, clonic convulsions, drowsiness, dysphoria/euphoria, death (if given rapidly in bolus).

CVS

Myocardial depression, decreased rate and force of contraction, sudden onset of ventricular fibrillation, cardiovascular collapse and death, in toxic levels.

Smooth Muscle

Relaxed vascular, gastrointestinal (GI) and bronchial smooth muscle and uterine muscle.

Neuromuscular Function

Affect transmission by blocking the nicotinic ACh receptors.

Local Anesthetics

Hypersensitivity

Allergic dermatitis, typical asthmatic attack, more common with ester type local anesthetic (LA).

Metabolism

Esters are hydrolyzed primarily by plasma esterase. Amide linked LAs are degraded by hepatic CYPs.

COCAINE

Local anesthetic (LA) actions and vasoconstriction (action due to inhibition of NE uptake). Cocaine hydrochloride 1%, 4%, 10% solutions are used for topical application. Associated euphoria leads to abuse potential. Cocaine should not be injected, as it is a protoplasmic poison. Causes tissue necrosis, stimulates vagal, vasomotor, chemoreceptor trigger zone (CTZ) and temperature-regulating center; bradycardia, increase BP, nausea, surface analgesia and vasoconstriction and increase body temperature may occur.

LIDOCAINE

- Most commonly used local anesthetic (LA).
- Total dose ranges from 500–750 mg. Maximum safe dose is 7 mg/kg with adrenaline, 3 mg/kg without adrenaline; itself causes local vasodilation.
- Lidocaine is formulated for topical, ophthalmic, mucosal and transdermal use.
- Combination of lidocaine (2.5%) and prilocaine (2.5%) formulated as 'Emla' used locally prior to venepuncture or skin grafting or infiltration of anesthetics.
- Relatively less toxic.
- Use: Topical, surface and infiltration anesthesia, nerve block, epidural, spinal, IV (Bier's block) regional block.
- Inadvertent venepuncture causes drowsiness, amnesia, cerebral depression; cardiorespiratory collapse may occur.
- Metabolized in liver, excreted via kidneys.
- Also used to treat ventricular fibrillation 100 mg (10 mL of a 1% solution) slow intravenously under cardiac monitoring.
- Drug used in spinal anesthesia is 5% and epidural anesthesia 1.2–5%, for infiltration 0.5%.
- Used as LA of intermediate duration of action.

BUPIVACAINE

- Potent amide local anesthetic (LA) with prolonged action.
- Produces more sensory than motor block.
- Used in providing analgesia during labor or postoperative period.
- More cardiotoxic than equi-effective doses of lignocaine; severe ventricular arrhythmia and myocardial depression can occur, due to slow dissociation of block of cardiac Na^+ channels.

- Recommended dose is 2 mg/kg. body weight. With adrenaline, dose is 2.5–3 mg/kg.
- Duration of action is about 3–5 hours for 0.5% solution with adrenaline.
- Bupivacaine-induced cardiac toxicity is difficult to treat and enhanced by acidosis, hypoxemia and hypercarbia.
  Prone to prolonged QTc interval and induces ventricular tachycardia or cardiac depression.

Local anesthetics suitable for injection:

Chloroprocaine	Ropivacaine
Articaine	Procaine
Mepivacaine	Tetracaine
Prilocaine	Others

Local anesthetics used to anesthetize mucous membranes or skin:

Dibucaine	Pramoxine
Dyclonine	Proparacaine (eye)

Local anesthetics with low solubility and hence directly applicable on wounds or ulcerated surfaces → Benzocaine.

Procaine	Fast onset of action
Chloroprocaine	
Prilocaine	Short duration
Lignocaine	
Mepivacaine	
Etidocaine	Onset of action moderate
Bupivacaine	long duration of action
Ropivacaine	
Levobupivacaine	

CLINICAL PREPARATION

Local anesthetics (LAs) are poorly soluble in water, presented as stable hydrochloride salts; pH varies from 5–6. Alkaline pH destabilizes local anesthetic, acidosis hinders the ionization and efficacy of a local anesthetic. Adrenaline in concentration of 1 in 200,000 or 1 in 400,000 is sometimes added to local anesthetic to decrease vascular absorption and toxicity.

Precautions to be Taken during Use

Syringe to be aspirated before injection to exclude puncture of blood vessel. Injection to be given slowly, especially in children, keeping vigilance on clinical signs and symptoms of hypersensitivity reactions or inadvertent IV injection.

An LA with adrenaline to be avoided in patients with IHD, uncontrolled hypertension, thyrotoxicosis or on tricyclic antidepressants/β blockers.

Procaine

- 0.25–1% for infiltration anesthesia.
- 1–2% for nerve block.

- Relatively nontoxic.
- Agent of choice in patients with malignant hyperreflexia.
- 5% is required for extradural block.
- Not used nowadays.

Chloroprocaine
- Rapid onset of action.
- Analgesia may disappear suddenly.
- Action lasts for 45 minutes.
- Used as 2-3% solution.
- Most acidic LA used.
- Paraplegia has been reported followed by intrathecal administration.
- Not used since then.

Tetracaine (Amethocaine)
- Used for topical or corneal analgesia.
- Highly lipid-soluble and potent.
- Slow to hydrolysis by pseudocholinesterase.
- Causes both surface and conduction block.
- Fast absorption can lead to toxicity.

Ropivacaine
- Newer bupivacaine congener.
- Equally long-acting.
- Less cardiotoxic.
- Blocks Aδ and C fibers > Aβ fibers (motor).
- Greater degree of separation between sensory and motor block.
- Continuous epidural ropivacaine is used in relieving postoperative pain and labor pain.

FEATURES OF AMIDE LA (TABLES 10.1 AND 10.2)
- Intense and long-lasting block.
- Bound to α_1 acid glycoprotein in plasma.
- Degraded by hepatic enzymes.
- Rarely cause hypersensitivity reactions.

Table 10.1: Comparative study of some local anesthetics.

Local anesthetic	Concentration used	Duration
Procaine	1–2%	½–1 hr
Lidocaine	0.5–2%	1–2 hrs
Tetracaine	0.25–0.5%	1½–4 hrs
Bupivacaine	0.25–0.5%	1½–3 hrs
Dibucaine	0.25–0.5%	1½–6 hrs

Table 10.2: Comparison of characteristics of local anesthetics.

Drug	Type	Concentration	Protein binding %	pKa	% of equivalent concentration	Onset	Duration	Maximum	Special comments
Cocaine	Ester	4% eye, 10–20% throat		8.7	1	Slow		Highly toxic	Koller first used it for eye operation, CNS stimulation, myocardial depression. Adrenaline should not be used
Lignocaine; Xylocaine	Amide	1–1.5% nerve block, 5% spinal, 1.2–5% epidermal	64	7.8	1	Rapid	60–120 mins	7 mg/kg. adrenaline, 3 mg without adrenaline, Medium toxic	Used in Rx in dysrhythmia, to attenuate hemodynamic effects of laryngoscopy
Bupivacaine; Sensorcaine, marcaine	Amide	0.5% epidermal, 0.25%, 0.75%	95	8.1	2–4	Modered	Long 3–6 hrs	Medium toxicity 2.5 mg/kg	Not recommended IV (Bier's) More cardiotoxic binds to myocardium. More sensory block than motor block
Etidocaine	Amide	1–1.5%	94	7.9	0.5	Quick	2–4 hrs	Medium toxicity 5 mg/kg	More profound motor block than sensory. Placental transfer is minimum, not used for topical/IV anesthesia

Contd...

Contd...

Drug	Type	Concentration	Protein binding %	pKa	% of equivalent concentration	Onset	Duration	Maximum	Special comments
Ropivacaine	Amide		94	8.1	0.25	Moderate	Long 4–8 hrs	150–200 mg. Medium toxicity	Propyl derivative of bupivacaine. Not used in topical/IV; used for regional block, epidural and spinal. Can cause differential sensory block (without motor block—useful in obstetrics)
Procaine	Ester	0.25–1%	58	8.9	2	Slow	Short	Low toxicity 500–1000 mg, 7 mg/kg body wt	CNS stimulation followed by depression; Quinidine like action on heart, should not be given with sulfonamides, hydrolyzed by plasma cholinesterase
Amethocaine	Ester	0.5% nerve block, 1% spinal	76	8.4	0.25	Slow	Long	Highly toxic	CNS stimulation followed by depression, vasodilation and quinidine like action, cardiotoxic

Onset time of blockade depends on the pka of the LA. LAs with low pka have fast onset of action compared with LA with higher pka, e.g. lignocaine (pka 7.6) faster onset than bupivacaine (pka 8.1). The pH at which the ionized and non-ionized form of a compound is present in equal amounts is defined as pka. For bases like LA, higher the pka, greater the ionized fraction.

MOLECULAR MECHANISM OF ACTION

Na^+ channel has an activation gate near the extracellular mouth and inactivation gate 'h' at the intracellular mouth. In the resting state, the activation gate is closed. Threshold depolarization of the membrane opens the activation gate to allow Na^+ ions to enter according to concentration gradient. Within a few seconds, the inactivation gate closes and ion flow ceases.

The LA receptor is located in the inner part of the Na^+ channel. The LA permeates through the axolemma in nonionized form and reionizes within the axoplasm and reaches the LA receptor. It is the cationic form which binds to the LA receptor and is accessible to the LA in the activated rather than in the resting state. After binding of the LA to the receptor; it stabilizes in inactive state and prevents further channel opening.

REGIONAL ANESTHESIA (TABLES 10.3 TO 10.5)

Loss of sensation in a region of the body due to action of local anesthetic agents on the nerves supplying the particular area, e.g. spinal anesthesia, epidural anesthesia.

Advantages

- The patient can be sedated and kept fully conscious as required.
- Sensory denervation of the operation site temporarily, relieving postoperative pain and responses to pain like tachycardia, increase in BP, increase in blood sugar, release of catecholamines and cortisol.

Table 10.3: Characteristics of regional anesthesia.

Characteristics	Subarachnoid	Epidural
Speed of onset	Very rapid	Delayed
Upper level of block	Variable	Satisfactory till T_4
Lower level of block	Satisfactory to S_4	Variable
Density of block	Profound	Variable
Duration of motor block	Prolonged	Usually not
Systemic absorption	Negligible	Substantial
Hypotension	Common	Variable
Shivering	Rare	Common
Dural puncture headache	Variable	Nil
Provision for postoperative analgesia	Nil	Ideal

Table 10.4: Complications of spinal anesthesia.

Immediate complications	Late sequelae
Hypotension	Postspinal headache
Nausea and vomiting	Backache
Headache	Urinary retention
Precordial discomfort	Meningitis
Limb paresthesia	Paralysis of VI cranial nerve
Difficulty in phonation	Other neurologic lesions
Inability to cough	Transient lesions of cauda equina radiculitis, ascending myelitis, transient transverse myelitis, adhesive arachnoiditis, paraplegia, anterior spinal artery syndrome (LMN paraplegia) without posterior involvement of postcolumn (Horner's syndrome)
Restlessness	
Hiccups	

Table 10.5: Complications of epidural anesthesia.

Immediate complications	Late sequelae
Inadequate block	Paraplegia
Hypotension	Anterior spinal artery syndrome
Nausea and vomiting	Backache
Total spinal	Intraocular hemorrhage
Toxicity of local anesthetic	Extradural abscess or hematoma
Prolonged analgesia	
Horner's syndrome	
Trigeminal nerve palsy	
Hiccups	

- Intraoperative blood loss is significantly less compared with general anesthesia.
- Postoperative morbidity due to cough, gastrointestinal stasis, pyrexia, immobility (causing deep vein thrombosis) is prevented.

Disadvantages

- *Inadequate anesthesia*: General blockade of T_4-S_5 is required, even then stimuli involving vagus nerve and lower surface of diaphragm are not relieved.
- *High spinal block*: Extensive block leading to decrease in forced expiratory volume (FEV_1), forced vital capacity (FVC), peak expiratory flow rate (PEFR) and pulmonary complications.

- Systemic toxicity due to absorption of local anesthetic.
- *Hypotension*: Sympathetic block, decrease in systemic vascular resistance (SVR), decrease in blood pressure (BP).
- Nausea/vomiting due to hypotension.
- *Shivering*: Seen more in epidural (treated by opioid).

Fetal and Neonatal Outcome in Cesarean Section done under Regional Anesthesia

Comparing regional and general anesthesia for CS, following assumptions have been made depending on neonatal acid–base status and Apgar score.
- Neonates born under general anesthesia are more likely to require resuscitation.
- Neonate born by regional anesthesia is more alert and responsive.
- Hypotension occurring during regional anesthesia appears to be of little consequence to neonatal outcome provided it is treated promptly and adequately.
- Time interval from incision to delivery seems to be less important in regional anesthesia.

Disadvantages of Spinal over Epidural Anesthesia

- Patient anxiety due to rapid onset.
- Greater chance of high block.
- Greater chance of hypotension.
- Higher incidence of vagal bradycardia.
- Dural puncture headache.

Prevention and Treatment of Hypotension due to Spinal Anesthesia

- Before operation, patient is turned fully to lateral position.
- Preloading with 500–1000 mL crystalloid.
- Vasopressor agents: Ephedrine 5 mg in incremental dosage is ideal.
- Other vasopressors: Phenylephrine 0.1 mg, methoxamine 0.5 mg, metaraminol 0.25 mg.
  First spinal analgesia done by Leonard Corning.
  First planned analgesia for surgery demonstrated by August Bier.

Contraindications for Subarachnoid Block and Extradural Anesthesia

- Bleeding diathesis.
- Sepsis close to the lumbar puncture (LP) site.
- Hypovolemia or shock or severe dehydration.
- Severe stenotic valvular disease.
- Pre-eclamptic toxemia (PET): Epidural can be used.
- Spinal deformity.
- Central nervous system (CNS) abnormality.

Points to Note:
- In spinal block, sympathetic fibers are blocked 2-3 segments higher than sensory fiber.
- In spinal block, difference between sensory and motor block is slight (2 segments); while in epidural block, difference in level is greater.
- Order of block of NV fibers—
    i. Autonomic preganglionic B fibers
    ii. Temperature fibers—cold before warm
    iii. Pin-prick fibers.
    iv. Deeper pain fibers
    v. Touch fibers
    vi. Deep pressure fibers
    vii. Somatic motor fibers
    viii. Vibratory sense and proprioceptive fibers.
- Returns in reverse order—sympathetic activity returns before senses.
- Local anesthetic acts on the nerve roots leaving the cord.
- Action depends on—accessibility via diffusion, lipid solubility, tissue blood flow, molecular weight, molecular shape and degree of ionization of the molecule.
- Blood pressure (BP) fall is usually seen within first 20 minutes after injection—sympathetic block causes dilatation of resistance capacitance vessels.
- Corrective measures for BP control should be considered if decrease in blood pressure is more than ⅓rd of preoperative value.
- Bradycardia is seen in high spinals (T_4-T_5); occurs due to vasovagal syndrome, block of cardiac sympathetic fibers (T_1-T_4).
- Differential nerve block occurs due to block of smaller fibers by weaker concentration.
- Blockade of sympathetic supply to heart leads to decrease in cardiac output, while that of adrenals lead to decrease in catecholamine release.
- Motor blockade to roots (C_{3-5}) of phrenic nerve causes apnea, decrease in vital capacity (VC), decrease in expiratory reserve volume (ERV) in high spinal; O_2 should be given.
- Higher parasympathetic activity in gut leads to constricted gut with increased peristaltic activity but sphincters are relaxed. Nausea and vomiting may occur.
- Decrease in blood circulation to liver and kidneys.
- Spinal block suppresses the hyperglycemic response to surgery and stress. Suppresses ADH increase in response to surgery.
- The response to insulin is augmented.
- Epidural anesthesia causes shivering because it is temperature sensitive (thermal sensor); large veins act as heat exchangers.
- Spinal needle selection = 22-26G. Quincke spinal needle facing laterally will minimize spinal headache.
- Drug should be introduced at the rate of 1 mL/5 sec.
- Vasoconstrictors are seldom used in spinal anesthesia for fear of compromise in blood supply to cord.

Note (Evidence based):
- Epidural anesthesia is better than parenteral opioids in relieving postoperative pain after major surgery and reduces the incidence of postoperative pneumonia.
- Clonidine increases the duration of regional block by about 2 hours but carries the risk of hypotension, bradycardia and sedation.

Factors Affecting Spread
- Dose of drug injected—most important.
- Volume of fluid injected.
- Specific gravity of solution—basicity compared to CSF; if 5-8% glucose is added it becomes hyperbaric.
- Position of patient during injection and after (lowest point of thoracic curve is T_5) the block.
- Choice of interspace (minor factor).
- Speed of injection— rapid injection leading to high block.
- Patient profile—age, height and pregnancy.

Factors which do not Influence Height of Analgesia in Spinal Block
- Patient weight and sex.
- Direction of bevel edge of needle; composition of fluid and addition of vasoconstrictor.
  Duration of action depends on drug dose, drug used and whether vasoconstrictor is present or not.

Drugs Used for Spinal Analgesia
- Bupivacaine: 0.5% in volume of 3-4 mL. Duration 2-3 hours.
- Lignocaine: 2% plain, 5% in dextrose 7.5% in 2.5 mL of plain/1.5 mL of heavy. Duration 1 hour.
- Prilocaine: 5% solution in 5% dextrose, rapid onset of action.
- Amethocaine: 1% in dextrose, maximum 20 mg.
- Procaine 5%.
- Mepivacaine: 4% solution with 10% glucose. Duration 1 hour.
  Sterilization of set by γ-ray or autoclearing.

Postspinal Headache
- More common in young adults especially in obstetric patients.
- It may occur even after 2-7 days of lumbar puncture (LP) and may persist up to 6 weeks, usually 1-2 weeks.
- Characteristically worsens on sitting and standing.
- Pain is often occipital and associated with stiffness of neck, may be vertical/frontal with pain in orbit.
- May be due to leakage of cerebrospinal fluid (CSF) into the epidural space, average loss 10 mL/hr.

Treatment

Prophylactic—proper selection of the patient. Needle of smaller gauge to be used—Quincke 25 G. Tuohy needle with Huber point may be used for epidural block. Prevention of dehydration and avoiding straining. Avoid repeated puncture and enter by separating dural fibers and not by tearing.

Curative

Patient should be supine till the anesthetic effect wears off (24 hours). Frequent drinks (less than 3 liter a day), O_2 inhalation, analgesics, tight abdominal binder (increase in venous return), continuous drip of Hartman's solution by Catheter and extradural blood patch by removing 20 mL. of blood from patient and injecting it into his extradural space at the site of puncture.

Diagnostic Criteria of Postspinal Headache

It is different from any other headache experienced by the patient. It is worsened by sitting or standing, and has occipital and nuchal components. It is relieved by abdominal compression.

Spinal anesthesia cannot be performed above L_2 due to the presence of spinal cord which may be liable to injury. But epidural anesthesia can be performed at any level, the site being guided by the level to be blocked.

Mechanism of Postspinal Headache

Traction on pain sensitive structures within the cranial cavity due to seepage of CSF through the dural puncture site. Pain pathway for headache includes trigeminal nerve (NV) in the 2/3rd of head, glossopharyngeal vagus and upper cervical nerves in the posterior 1/3rd.

EPIDURAL BLOCK

- Equipment : 16-G Tuohy needle with Huber point.
- Rate of drug infusion - 10 mL/min.
- For catheterization 2-3 cm of catheter should be inside.

Site of Action
- Nerve roots in epidural space.
- Nerve roots in paravertebral space.
- Nerve roots in subarachnoid space after diffusion.
- Diffusion into subperineural and subpial spaces.

Factors Influencing Spread
- Volume of drug.
- Age of patient.
- Force of injection.
- Amount of drug used.
- Level of injection.

- Length of vertebral column.
- Pregnancy or abdominal tumors.
- Concentration of local anesthetic.
- Presence of diabetes or vaso-occlusive diseases.

Factors Affecting Onset
- Concentration of drug in the solution.
- Presence of vasoconstrictor.

Factors Affecting Duration
- Type of drug.
- Concentration of drug.
- Presence of vasoconstrictor.

Total Spinal Anesthesia

This may occur if a large volume of drug (even 10 mL) intended for epidural anesthesia is (by mistaken) injected into the subarachnoid space. It usually occurs soon after administration may be delayed for 30–45 minutes.

Clinical features—within 3 minutes, there is profound hypotension, apnea, dilated pupils, loss of consciousness, paralysis of legs; should arouse suspicion. There is grave danger of death from asphyxia unless promptly managed.

Management

Turn patient to supine position. Ventilate the lungs, elevate the legs, inject pressor drug, administer IV fluid. Later intubation followed by intermittent positive pressure ventilation (IPPV) till normal breathing returns. Surgery can be carried on as patient reverts in an hour. Unpleasant sequelae are unlikely.

Agents Used for Epidural

Lignocaine 1.5–2% with or without 1.200,000 adrenaline. Bupivacaine 0.25%, 0.5%, 0.75%, addition of adrenaline prolongs duration of action.

Therapeutic Use of Epidural Injection

- Postoperative pain relief.
- Management of closed chest injury.
- Eclampsia.
- Control of labor pain.
- Control of chronic pain due to cancer.
- Acute vaso-occlusive disease.

CHAPTER 11

Drugs Used in Nausea and Vomiting

INTRODUCTION

- Nausea and vomiting are unpleasant feelings associated with a variety of factors like chemotherapeutic drugs, disease conditions, motion sickness even ghastly sight, unpleasant odor, fear or pain.
- Two brainstem centers, the chemoreceptor trigger zone (CTZ) in area postrema and the VC (vomiting center) in the lateral reticular formation of medulla, are primarily responsible.
- The CTZ situated outside the blood-brain barrier (BBB) is stimulated by variety of factors like cytotoxic drugs, infection, radiation and GI irritation via $5HT_3$, D_2, H_1, µ, and M receptors.
- The VC is stimulated by various afferent stimuli from cerebral cortex (sight, odor, pain, fear), vestibular (due to rotational movement or ototoxic drugs), cerebellum or peripheral stimuli from oropharynx or GI, via D_2, $5HT_3$, M and H receptors.
- Drugs which may induce vomiting are emetine, morphine, cytotoxic drugs or chemotherapeutic agents, digitalis, apomorphine, ergot alkaloids.
- Thus antiemetic drugs act primarily by inhibiting the receptors at CTZ or VC or the periphery either by obliterating the efferent impulses from the brainstem or by increasing lower esophageal sphincteric tone and those affecting GI motility are also known as prokinetic agents.

CLASSIFICATION (FIG. 11.1)

- *D_2 receptor antagonists*: Metoclopramide and domperidone.
- *Anticholinergics*: Hyoscine and dicyclomine.
- *Antihistamines*: Meclizine, cyclizine and cinnarizine
  - Other phenothiazines: Promethazine, diphenhydramine and doxylamine
- *$5HT_3$ receptor blockers*: Ondansetron, granisetron and dolasetron.
- *Prokinetic agents*: Cisapride, mosapride and prucalopride.

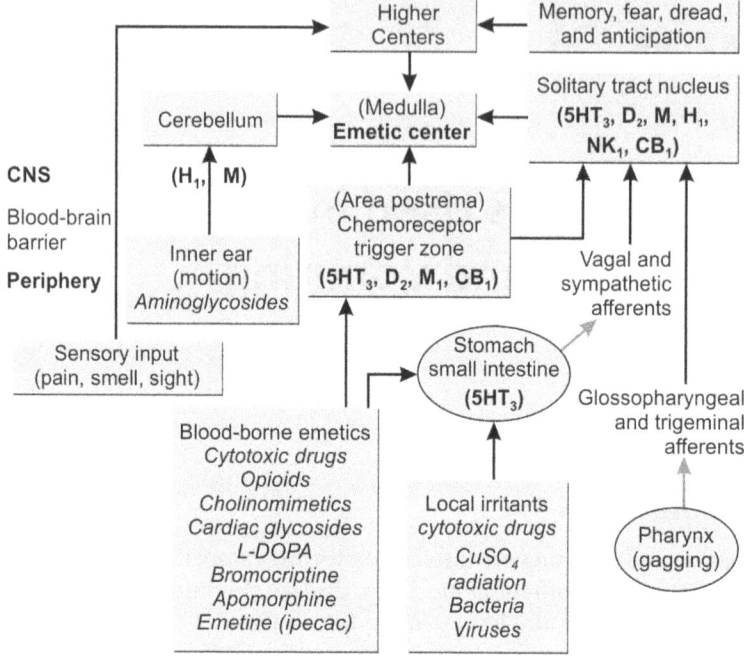

Figure 11.1: Mechanism of vomiting.

- Butyrophenones: Droperidol and haloperidol.
- Motilides: Erythromycin and other macrolides.
- Newer drugs
  - Substance P/Neurokinin – 1 – blocker–aprepitant.
  - CCK-A receptor antagonist—dexloxiglumide.
  - Somatostatin analogue—octreotide, clonidine.
  - Cannabinoids—dronabinol, nabilone.
- Adjuvant antiemetics
  - Benzodiazepines, e.g. alprazolam and lorazepam, corticosteroids, e.g. dexamethasone.

Metoclopramide

Chemically related to procainamide.

Mode of action: Central; inhibits $5HT_3$ receptor at CTZ. Peripheral; increase gastric emptying, increase esophageal (LES) tone, $5HT_4$ agonism in GIT (enhance ACh release from myenteric plexus).

Indications of use: Effective antiemetic, to induce gastric emptying, dyspepsia and GERD.

Can be used orally, parenterally or rectally.

Contraindications: Hepatic insufficiency, <20 years age, gastric obstruction or pregnancy, parkinsonism, pheochromocytoma.

Adverse effects: EPS (young people < 20 years susceptible), parkinsonism like signs and symptons: Dizziness, drowsiness, prolactin release → galactorrhea, gynecomastia.

Dose: 0.15–0.3 mg/kg, oral dose is 10 mg.

Domperidone

Structurally related to haloperidol penetrates BBB poorly; acts only on the CTZ which is outside the BBB, so EPS/hyperprolactinemia is rare.

Action: Acts as D_2 receptor antagonists at CNS and periphery.

Indication: Nausea and vomiting due to cytotoxic drugs or dopaminergic agonists, postoperative nausea, dopa-induced vomiting.

Contraindication: Pregnancy, motion sickness, GI obstruction.

Dose: 10 mg orally thrice daily.

Adverse effects: Increase prolactin secretion → hyperprolactinemia, galactorrhea, gynecomastia, rash.

Preferred to metoclopramide due to less adverse effects though antiemetic action is less compared to metoclopramide.

$5HT_3$ Receptor Antagonists

$5HT_3$ receptors in GI tract activate the visceral afferent sensory neurons in GI tract and carry impulses to spinal cord and CNS. Blocking peripheral $5HT_3$ receptors inhibit the unpleasant sensations like nausea, vomiting, pain and bloating; blocking of enteric cholinergic neurons inhibit colonic motility. Blockade of central $5HT_3$ receptors depresses the central responses to peripheral stimuli. Hence, they are effective in vomiting due to various etiology especially chemotherapy-induced vomiting; moreover, they enhance GI motility.

Ondansetron

- Prototype $5HT_3$ antagonist.
- Orally administered, ondansetron has bioavailability of 60–70%.
- Undergoes first pass hepatic metabolism.
- Metabolized in liver by CYP1A2, CYP2D6, CYP3A and excreted via kidney.
- Dose adjustments are required in hepatic insufficiency.
- t½ is about 4–12 hours.

Uses
- Vomiting due to chemotherapeutic drugs.
- Radiation-induced vomiting.
- Postoperative nausea and vomiting.
- During therapy of other emetogenic drugs.
- Used preoperatively as preanesthetic medication.
- Vomiting associated with drug overdoses.
- Uremia/neurological injury-associated vomiting.

Adverse effects
- More or less well tolerated; no significant drug interactions.
- Headache and dizziness.
- Constipation/diarrhea.
- Hypersensitive reactions followed by IV administration.

Dose: 4–8 mg IV slowly over 15 minutes repeated twice at an interval of 4 hours.

Orally: 8 mg twice daily.

Granisetron

- 10–15 times more potent than ondansetron.
- Longer half-life: 8–12 hours.
- Weak $5HT_4$ blocking action of ondansetron is absent with granisetron.
- More effective as antiemetogenic; effective in twice daily dosing.

Dose: 10 µg/kg IV repeated at 12 hourly interval; side effects similar to ondansetron, orally 1–2 mg twice daily.

Palonosetron

- Excellent oral absorption.
- Metabolized in liver, excreted via kidney.
- t½—40 hours.
- Onset of action 24 hours.
- Popular as antiemetic in chemotherapy-induced vomiting.
- Side effects profile similar to ondansetron.

Alosetron

- $5HT_3$ antagonist approved for use in severe IBS, with diarrhea.
- Highly potent.
- Selective blocker of $5HT_3$ receptor.
- Rapid absorption, bioavailability (BA) of 50–60%.
- Plasma t½: 1.5 hours.
- Longer duration of action as it binds to receptors with higher affinity and dissociates more slowly compared to other $5HT_3$ antagonists.
- Metabolized by CYP450 enzymes excreted via kidney.

Uses: Irritable bowel syndrome (IBS) associated with diarrhea associated abdominal pain, cramp, urgency. Other idiopathic diarrhea.
- Side effects—Excellent safely profile, constipation, rarely ischemic colitis.

Anticholinergics and Antihistaminics

Indications: Motion sickness, vomiting due to neoplastic disease, opioid-induced vomiting, postoperative vomiting, extrapyramidal symptoms (EPS) due to metoclopramide.

Hyoscine

- Anticholinergic commonly used in treatment of motion sickness.
- Short duration of action.
- Blocks transmission of impulse from vestibular apparatus to vomiting center.
- Produces sedation and dryness of mouth.
- Useful for premedication due to its antisecretory, sedative and anti-emetic action.
- Can be used orally, IM, as transdermal patch applied behind the pinna.
- Adverse effects minimum, e.g. sedation and dryness of mouth.
- Dose—0.2–0.4 mg oral/IM.

Dicyclomine

- Anticholinergic used in the treatment or prophylaxis of morning sickness due to absence of teratogenic effects.
- Can also be used to prevent motion sickness.
- Available as 10–20 mg oral tablet.

Doxylamine

- Antihistaminic (H_1 receptor blocker) with prominent anticholinergic activity.
- Its antiemetic action is due to its antihistaminic, anticholinergic and sedative property.
- Marketed in combination with pyridoxine in the treatment and prophylaxis of morning sickness.
- Side effect: Drowsiness, vertigo and dry mouth.
- Dose: 10–20 mg orally.

Cyclizine and Meclizine

Antihistaminics with less anticholinergic and sedative action. Used for motion sickness, meclizine with long half-life can be used for sea-sickness.

Cinnarizine

Has additional antivertigo action as it also inhibits Ca^{+2} influx from endolymph inhibiting vestibular reflexes. Can be used in motion sickness due to its antihistaminic and anticholinergic action.

Prokinetic Agents

Medications which enhance coordinated GI motility and help in transition of material in GIT, stimulating motor neurons by increasing release of excitatory neurotransmission at nerve-muscle junction. They thereby:
- Increase lower esophageal sphincter tone
- Increase gastric emptying
- Increase intestinal peristalsis

without altering normal physiology

Prokinetic drugs are metoclopramide, domperidone, cisapride, mosapride, renzapride and motilides.

Indication: Postoperative paralytic ileus, gastroparesis and chronic idiopathic constipation.

Cisapride

- Prokinetic agent without any antiemetic activity.
- Major action is as agonists on $5HT_4$ receptors and antagonistic action on $5HT_3$ receptors, increase ACh release and GI stimulatory activity; at the same time suppressing the inhibitory effects on myenteric plexus respectively.
- Oral bioavailability of 33%, metabolized in the liver by CYP3A4 enzymes; t½ of 10 hours.
- Uses: GERD, impaired gastric emptying or gastroparesis, nonulcer dyspepsia.
- Adverse effects: Diarrhea, abdominal cramps, dizziness, increase in hepatic enzymes. At high concentration, cisapride may prolong QTc interval and induce torsades de pointes or ventricular arrhythmia. Due to its life-threatening adverse effects, cisapride has been withdrawn from the market.
- Dose: 10–20 mg thrice daily.

Mosapride

$5HT_4$ agonist with mild antagonistic action at $5HT_3$ receptor. It does not cause prolongation of QT interval, hence safe. Has no antiemetic action.
- Uses: GERD, gastroparesis and nonulcer dyspepsia.
- Dose: 5 mg thrice daily.

Prucalopride

- Benzofuran derivative.
- $5HT_4$ agonistic activity, facilitating ACh activity.
- Stimulates motility of small intestine and colon without affecting gastric emptying.
- Use: Chronic idiopathic constipation.
- Dose: 2–4 mg. orally.

Others

Motilides: Macrolide antibiotics especially erythromycin bind to motilin receptors of gastrointestinal tract (GIT) causing increased motility though tolerance develops rapidly. Motilin is a peptide hormone found in M-cells of GIT and some enterochromaffin cells of small gut; motilin receptors are present in the smooth muscles of GIT.
- *Action*: Increase lower esophageal sphincter pressure, stimulates gastric and intestinal motility. No action is seen in colon.
- *Use*: Diabetic gastroparesis, paralytic ileus and GI dysmotility in scleroderma.

- *Dose*: Erythromycin 3 mg/kg IV or 200-250 mg orally thrice daily.
- *Other drugs used*: Macrolide antibiotics like azithromycin, clarithromycin, mitemcinal (nonantibiotic macrolide).

Sincalide: C-terminal peptide of cholecystokinin (CCK) used in stimulating gallbladder (GB) and pancreas. It can also be used to increase the transit time of barium through small bowel during diagnostic testing.

Dexloxiglumide
- CCK receptor antagonist used in improving gastric emptying.
- Use: Gastroparesis, constipation dominant irritable bowel syndrome (IBS).

Other Drugs used in GI Motility Disorders
- Tegaserod: Serotonergic prokinetic drug, not available nowadays, used in constipation predominant irritable bowel syndrome (IBS).
- Clonidine: Beneficial in gastroparesis.
- Octreotide acetate: Somatostatin analogue used in patients with intestinal dysmotility.

Others

- *Dronabinol*
  - Naturally occurring cannabinoid extracted from cannabis sativa.
  - Useful prophylactic in cancer chemotherapy vomiting.
  - Stimulates appetite.
  - Given 1-3 hours before chemotherapy, then 2-4 hours afterward for 4-6 doses.
  - Adverse effect: prominent sympathomimetic activity.
- *Dexamethasone*: Useful in nausea in patients with widespread cancer. Acts by suppressing peritumoral inflammation and blocking the action of PGs.
- *Benzodiazepines*: By relieving anxiety, decrease anticipatory component of nausea. Benefit is seen due to anxiolytic, sedative and amnesic properties.
- *Substance P antagonists*: Antagonists of NK_1 receptors for substance P, e.g. aprepitant have antiemetic effects in the delayed phase of nausea induced by cytotoxic agents like cisplatin (2-5 days following chemotherapy). Substance P is in vagal afferent fibers innervating Substantia nigra (STN) and area postrema.
  - Aprepitant is administered along with dexamethasone and palonosetron. Orally administered, it undergoes metabolism itself as well as induces CYP3A4 enzymes and causes drug interaction.
  - *Side effects*: Fatigue, constipation.
  - *Indication*: Vomiting due to chemotherapy agents.
  - *Point to note (Evidence based)*: Postoperative nausea prophylaxis should target inclusion of dexamethasone, droperidol and a $5HT_3$ antagonist.

COMPARATIVE STUDY OF COMMONLY USED DRUGS

Drug; (Generic and trade name)	Dose and dosage form	Indications	Remarks
Hyoscine	0.2–0.4 mg SOS; Oral tab, IM inj, transdermal patch	Motion sickness, preanesthetic medication	Poor antiemetic of other etiologies; anticholinergic adverse effects
Doxylamine: Doxinate, gravidox	10–20 mg SOS; oral tablet	Vomiting of pregnancy	Drowsiness, vertigo
Meclizine: Diligan, pregnidoxin	12.5 mg, 25 mg	Motion sickness, sea sickness	Antihistaminic with less anticholinergic action
Metoclopramide: Perinorm, Reglan	0.1–0.8 mg/kg/day; 10 mg tab, 5 mg/mL inj	Nausea, vomiting, GI dysmotility	EPS, use to be avoided in children
Domperidone: Domstal, domperon	0.2–0.4 mg/kg/dose; 10–20 mg TDS/QDS	Nausea, vomiting of any cause	Dry mouth, headache, rashes
Mosapride: Moza, mopride, mozasef	2.5–5 mg tablet thrice daily	Nonulcer dyspepsia, GERD	May cause QT prolongation, cardiac arrhythmias
Itopride: Itoflux, ganaton, itokine	50 mg tablet; thrice daily before meals	GI motility disorders	Devoid of drug interactions and EPS
Ondansetron: Emeset, osetron, ondy	8 mg IV over 15 min, 4–8 mg IV 8 mg orally BD	Vomiting due to drugs, chemotherapy, radiotherapy	Dose adjustment required in hepatic dysfunction
Granisetron: Graniset, granicip, grandem	1–3 mg 12 hourly 1/2 mg tab, 1 mg/mL inj	Vomiting of chemotherapy, PONV	10 times more potent than ondansetron

CHAPTER 12

Drugs Used in Peptic Ulcer Disease

INTRODUCTION

Peptic ulcer disease occurs due to disbalance between gastric acid secretion and mucosal defence mechanism. Stomach secretes about 25 L of gastric juice comprising primarily of HCl, secreted from parietal/oxyntic cells and pepsinogen from chief-peptic cells. Mucus and HCO_3 secreted throughout the gastric mucosa is controlled by PGs E_2 and I_2.

Gastric acid secretion is under the control of neuronal stimulation releasing ACh, histamine and endocrine factors like gastrin. The terminal enzyme responsible for H^+ ion secretion from the gastric parietal cell is the H^+K^+ATPase (proton pump) which is stimulated by ACh (M_3 receptor), histamine (H_2 receptor) and gastrin (CCK_2 receptor) at the basolateral part of the parietal cell. Some receptors are also present on enterochromaffin like cells which release histamine. Somatostatin secreted by antral D cells inhibit gastric acid secretion.

Principal pathological conditions which are associated with increased acid production are (i) duodenal and gastric ulcer, (ii) reflex esophagitis, and (iii) Zollinger–Ellison syndrome.

Helicobacter pylori a gram-negative bacillus is said to be responsible for chronic gastritis/duodenal ulcer.

CLASSIFICATION (TABLE 12.1)

Drugs used in peptic ulcer can be classified as:
- Neutralization of gastric acid by antacids; systemic antacid, e.g. $NaHCO_3$ and Na-citrate; Nonsystemic antacid, e.g. Mg $(OH)_2$, Al $(OH)_3$, magnesium trisilicate magaldrate.
- Reduction of gastric acid secretion: Proton pump inhibitors—e.g. pantoprazole, omeprazole, H_2 antagonists/antihistaminics—cimetidine, famotidine, roxatidine.
    Anticholinergics: M_2 antagonists—pirenzepine, propantheline, oxyphenonium.

Table 12.1: Comparative study of commonly used drugs.

Drug; (Generic and trade name)	Dose	Dosage form	Comments
Ranitidine: Rantac, zinetac, aciloc	150 mg BD or 300 mg at BT, 50 mg IM/slow IV	150 mg tablet, 50 mg/2 mL inj	Prophylaxis and treatment of peptic ulcer, stress ulcers, gastrinoma
Famotidine: Famtac, famocid, topcid	20 mg BD or 40 mg at BT	20 mg tab, 40 mg tab, 20 mg/2mL inj	ZE syndrome, aspiration pneumonia
Roxatidine Rotane	75 mg BD or 150 mg at BT	75 mg, 150 mg SR tablet	Peptic ulcer, GERD, ZE syndrome, stress ulcer
Pantoprazole; Pantodac, Pantocid	40 mg OD	20 mg or 40 mg SR tablet	Peptic ulcer, stress ulcer prophylaxis
Lansoprazole	15–30 mg OD	15 mg, 30 mg tab	Inhibition of $H^+ K^+$ AT-Pase is partly reversible
Rabeprazole	20 mg OD	10 mg, 20 mg tab	Fastest acid suppression
Sodium citrate			1 g neutralizes 10 mEq HCl
Aluminum hydroxide: Aludrox		0.84 g tab, 0.6 g/10 mL suspension	Hypophosphatemia can occur on regular use. 1 g neutralizes 1–2.5 mEq HCl

   Prostaglandin analogs: Misoprostol, enprostil and rioprostil (used in NSAID-induced ulcer).
- Ulcer protectives: Sucralfate, colloidal bismuth subcitrate.
- Ulcer healing: Carbenoxolone sodium.
- Anti-*H. pylori* drugs: Amoxycillin, clarithromycin, tinidazole and tetracycline.

H_2 ANTAGONISTS

Highly selective do not affect H_1 or H_3 receptor. Inhibit action of histamine at all H_2 receptors, specially gastric acid secretion. Competitive antagonists—cimetidine, ranitidine, roxatidine.

Competitive noncompetitive antagonists, e.g. famotidine, and non-competitive antagonist, e.g. loxatidine.

Pharmacokinetics
- Well-absorbed orally, may be given by IM/IV route; absorption increased by food and decreased by antacids.
- Bioavailability—60–80%.
- First-pass hepatic metabolism; Nizatidine has little first pass metabolism – BA is 100%.
- Metabolized in liver.
- Crosses placenta, secreted in milk.

- Hydrophillic, 2/3rd excreted unchanged in urine and bile, rest are oxidized.
- Elimination t½ 2–3 hours.
- Dose to be decreased in renal compromised patients.

Pharmacodynamics
- Decreased gastric secretion in all the phases.
- Uterine relaxation and bronchial relaxation is there.
- Fall in blood pressure (BP), specially late phase response seen in high doses.
- Most prominent action is on basal acid output, but volume, pepsin content and intrinsic factor secretion are also reduced (Vitamin B_{12} absorption is not interfered).
- Ranitidine, nizatidine may stimulate gastrointestinal (GI) motility.

Adverse Effects
- Headache, drowsiness, fatigue, dry mouth, bowel upset, diarrhea, muscle pain, transient rashes and fever may occur.
- IV bolus injection may cause bradycardia, arrhythmias and cardiac arrest.
- Transient neutropenia and transient increase of aminotransferases.
- Cimetidine has antiandrogenic action by decreasing testosterone binding to receptor, increasing plasma prolactin, inhibits degradation of estradiol by liver and causes gynecomastia, impotence, lack of libido.

Uses
(i) Peptic ulcer, (ii) Stress ulcers and gastritis, (iii) ZE syndrome, (iv) GERD, (v) Prophylaxis against aspiration preumonia (vi) Others, e.g. urticaria (in addition to H_1 antihistaininics).
- Ranitidine—5 times as potent as cimetidine. Hepatic injury, CNS effects and hematological effects are rare, lesser incidence of side effect. Administered 300 mg orally at bed time as nocturnal dose. Administered 50 mg IM/IV twice daily.
- Cimetidine inhibits CYP450 and inhibits metabolism of theophylline, phenytoin, phenobarbitone, warfarin, digoxin, quinidine, nifedipine, mexiletine, propranolol and diazepam.
- Famotidine (20 mg) BD—5–8 times more potent than ranitidine. Minimum side effects and drug interactions. More useful in Zollinger-Ellison (ZE) syndrome and prevention of aspiration pneumonia.
- Nizatidine (150 mg)—little first-pass metabolism, bioavailability almost 100%. Disadvantage—drug interactions, development of tolerance and hypergastrinemia.

PROTON PUMP INHIBITORS

These are highly efficacious acid inhibiting agents. These have structural similarity to H_2 receptor blockers but have different mechanisms of action.

These suppress gastric acid secretions in a dose-dependent manner by reacting covalently with the -SH group of H^+ K^+ ATPase enzyme and inactivating it irreversibly.

Pharmacokinetics

- They are administered as inactive prodrugs.
- As the prodrug is acid lable they are provided as acid resistant enteric-coated tablets, which dissolve in alkaline pH.
- Prodrug is rapidly protonated and concentrated in the parietal cell canaliculi, of stomach after absorption.
- Bioavailability is reduced by food, hence to be taken ideally 30 minutes before a meal.
- Duration of acid inhibition lasts for 24 hours.
- Rapid first-pass metabolism and systemic hepatic metabolism with negligible renal clearance.
- Also inhibits carbonic anhydrase in gastric mucosa.
- Oral absorption is 50%, H^+K^+ATPase inhibition occurs in 1 hour, reaches maximum in 2 hours, and lasts 3 days. Enzyme takes 18 hours to regenerate.
- Avoid long-term use of proton pump inhibitors due to chance of compensatory hypergastrinemia. It may take 2-5 days to achieve 70% inhibition of proton pump in once daily dosing.

Adverse Effects

- Adverse effects are minimum with headache, myopathy, arthralgia, nausea, abdominal pain, loose stools.
- Rashes, leukopenia and hepatic dysfunction is rare.
- Increase in chance of enteric infections, e.g. *Salmonella*, and hyper-gastrinemia on prolonged use.
- Esomeprazole-S-enantiomer of omeprazole. It has got 50-89% bioavailability. It has got better control of pH than omeprazole.
- *Lansoprazole*: It has got higher oral bioavailability (80-90%) and faster onset of action. Dose to be reduced in the case of liver disease.
- *Pantoprazole*: Similar potency but more acid stable, available for IV infusion, specially in bleeding peptic ulcer. Dose 40 mg daily × 10 days.
- *Rabeprazole*: It claims to cause fastest acid suppression, potency and efficacy similar to omeprazole.

Drug Interactions

Bioavailabity of ketoconazole, ampicillin esters, iron salts altered due to decrease in pH.

PROSTAGLANDIN ANALOGS

Misoprostol or methyl analog of PGE_1, has both acid inhibitory and mucosal protective properties. It stimulates mucus and bicarbonate secretion and enhance mucosal blood flow. It binds to prostaglandin receptor of parietal cells.

Misoprostol is rapidly absorbed; undergoes extensive first-pass metabolism to form active metabolite. Inhibition of acid secretion occurs in 30 minutes, peaks in 60–90 minutes, lasts for 3 hours. Food and antacids decrease the rate of absorption production and causing modest acid inhibition. It inhibits acid output, dose dependently, 200 µg reducing basal secretion by 90% and stimulated secretion by 80%.

Uses
NSAID-induced peptic ulcer.

Adverse Effects
The effects are diarrhea, cramping, abdominal pain, stimulates uterine contractions, and it should not be used during pregnancy. Dose 200 µg four times daily.

SUCRALFATE
It is a salt of sucrose complexed to sulfated aluminum hydroxide.

Mechanism of Action
In water or acidic solutions it forms a viscous tenacious paste that binds selectively to ulcers or erosions for up to 6 hours, forming a physical barrier. It may also bind epithelial growth factor and fibroblast growth factor, enhancing mucosal repair.

Dose
1 g QDS at least 1 hour before meals four times daily.

Uses
Healing of duodenal ulcers, oral mucositis, rectal ulcer, radiation proctitis and preventing bleeding from stress ulcers.

Side Effects
Constipation occurs in 2% due to aluminum salt. No side effect as it is not absorbed. It should not be used for prolonged periods in renal insufficiency and is not useful in NSAID-induced ulcers.

Drug Interactions
Affects absorption of phenytoin, digoxin, cimetidine, fluoroquinolones and ketoconazole.

COLLOIDAL BISMUTH
Bismuth subsalicylate undergoes rapid dissociation within the stomach, allowing absorption of salicylate. 99% of bismuth appears in the stool. Although minimal less than 1% bismuth is absorbed. It has slow renal excretion and salicylate is excreted in urine.

Mechanism of Action

It heals ulcer by:
- Increase in secretion of mucus and bicarbonate through stimulation of mucosal PGE_2.
- Colloidal bismuth subsalicylate (CBS) and mucus form a glycoprotein—bicomplex, which coats the ulcer and acts as a diffusion barrier to gastric acid.
- Detaches *H. pylori* from the surface of mucosa and directly kills this organism.

Dosage

120 mg half an hour before 3 major meals.

Side Effects

Causes diarrhea, headache and dizziness. Prolonged use has the potential to cause osteodystropy and encephalopathy and darkening of tongue.

Uses

Dyspepsia, prevention of traveler's diarrhea, eradication of *H. pylori* infection. Prolonged use of bismuth agents should be avoided in patients with renal insufficiency.

ANTACIDS

They were mainstay of treatment until the advent of H_2 blockers and $H^+K^+ATPase$ pump inhibitors.

Mechanism of Action

Antacids are weak bases that react with gastric HCl to form salt and water; hence decrease in intragastric acidity. They may also promote mucosal defence mechanism through stimulation of mucosal PG production.

Agents used Commonly with Adverse Effects

- *Magnesium hydroxide*: Osmotic diarrhea.
- *Aluminum hydroxide*: Constipation.
- *Sodium bicarbonate*: Gastric distension, belching metabolic alkalosis and fluid retention.
- *Calcium carbonate*: Less soluble, belching and metabolic alkalosis with dairy products. Increased doses produce renal insufficiency, hypercalcemia and metabolic alkalosis (milk alkali syndrome).

Drug Interactions

Antacid affects absorption of—tetracyclines, fluoroquinolones, itraconazole, ketoconazole, iron, phenothiazines, digoxin, indomethacin and fat-soluble vitamins.

The relative efficacy of antacids is expressed as milliequivelent of acid neutralization. According to FDA antacids should have a neutralizing capacity of at least 5 mEq/dose. Administered as suspension or chewable tablets.

CHAPTER 13

Drugs Used in Treatment of Asthma

DRUGS FOR BRONCHIAL ASTHMA

DEFINITION

The American Thoracic Society defines asthma as "a disease characterized by an increased responsiveness of the trachea and bronchi to various stimuli and manifested by a widespread narrowing of the airways that changes in severity either spontaneously or as a result of the treatment."

- *Types*: Intrinsic, extrinsic and unspecified.
- *Incidence*: About 5% of general population, 10% in children, 5% in adults. Overall mortality is about 20 million persons.
- *Etiology*: URTI, stress, exercise, allergen, industrial pollutants, environmental pollutants, e.g. ozone, NO_2 and SO_2.
- *Drugs*: NSAIDs, β blockers, aspirin, coloring agents like tartrazine.
- *Genetic predisposition*: ADAM 37 gene is strongly associated.
- *Pathophysiology*: The pathophysiologic hallmark of asthma is a reduction in airway brought about by vascular congestion, edema of bronchial wall, contraction of smooth muscles brought about by inflammation. Inflammation of bronchial asthma differs from inflammation found in other conditions, by hyper-reactivity.
- *Inflammation is associated with*:
  – Increase in inflammatory cells and their activation.
  – Release of a large number of inflammatory mediators like histamine, PG, leukotrienes, interleukins, synthesis of postinflammatory cytokines, increase in IgE.

Thus, the above pathophysiology predicts that a drug affecting only one mediator is unlikely to be of any substantial benefit.

CLASSIFICATION OF DRUGS USED IN BRONCHIAL ASTHMA (TABLES 13.1 AND 13.2)

I. *Bronchodilators (Fig. 13.1)*:
   A. Sympathomimetics: Adrenaline (α, β), ephedrine (α, β) and isoprenaline (β). Selective β_2 agonists—salbutamol, terbutaline, bambuterol, salmeterol, formoterol.
   B. Methylxanthines: Theophylline and aminophylline.
   C. Anticholinergics: Atropine methonitrate, ipratropium bromide and tiotropium bromide.
II. *Corticosteroids*:
   A. Systemic: Hydrocortisone, prednisolone and others.
   B. Inhalational: Beclomethasone dipropionate, budesonide, fluticasone propionate, flunisolide.

Table 13.1: Treatment module of various grades of asthma.

1.	Mild intermittent; SaO_2 > 95%, $PaCO_2$ < 42 mm Hg	Symptoms ≤ 2/week FEV_1/ PEF ≥ 80% predicted PEF variability ≤ 20%	Nighttime symptoms ≤ 2 times/ month. Exacerbations brief	Short-acting bronchodilation. Inhaled β_2 agonists. If required β_2 agonists > 2 times/week	Long-term therapy?
2.	Mild persistent; SaO_2— 91–95% $PaCO_2$ < 42 mm Hg	Symptoms > 2 times/week but < 1 time/ day. FEV_1/ PEF > 80% predicted PEF variability ≥ 20–30%	Nighttime symptoms > 2 times/ month. Exacerbations may affect activity	*Quick relief* Inhaled β_2 agonists. Intensity of treatment depends on severity of symptoms	Long-term control, inhaled corticosteroids or cromolyn or nedocromil
3.	Moderate persistent; SaO_2 < 91% $PaCO_2$ ≥ 42 mm Hg	*Daily symptoms* Daily use of β_2 agonist (short-acting) FEV_2/ PEF > 60–80%, PEF variability > 30%	*Nighttime symptoms* > 1 time/ week. Exacerbations ≥ 2 times/week	*Quick relief* Inhaled β_2 agonists. Intensity depends on severity	Long-term control; inhaled corticosteroids, long-acting bronchodilator
4.	Severe persistent; SaO_2 < 91% $PaCO_2$ ≥ 42 mm Hg	*Continual symptoms* Limited physical-activity, frequent exacerbations FEV_1 ≤ 60%, PEF variability > 30%	Nighttime symptoms are frequent. Exacerbations are frequent	*Quick relief* Inhaled β_2 agonists. Intensity of treatment depends on severity	Long-term control, inhaled corticosteroids, long-acting β_2 agonists, systemic or oral corticosteroids (not exceeding 60 mg/day)

Table 13.2: Comparison of anti-asthma drugs.

Drug; (Generic and trade name)	Dose	Dosage form	Indication	Comments
Salbutamol: Asthalin, ventorlin	0.1–0.4 mg/kg/dose 8 hourly oral, 4–6 µg/kg/dose SC, IM, IV	2 mg, 4 mg CR tab; 2–4 puffs 4–6 hourly in metered dose, inhaler also nebulizer	Mild to moderate asthma	Inhalational route preferable
Bambuterol; Bambudil, Bemlo	10–20 mg/day	10 mg, 20 mg tab, 5 mg/5 mL syrup	Maintenance therapy of asthma in adults	Prodrug of terbutaline
Theophylline	15–25 mg/kg/day 8 hourly		Severe asthma, when inhalation route not effective	Toxicity occurs if blood level ≥ 30 µg/mL
Aminophylline; Aminophylline	15–20 mg/kg/day	100 mg tab, 250 mg/10 mL inj	Severe bronchoconstriction, status asthmaticus	Can be given IV slowly but not IM/SC
Ipratropium bromide; Ipravent	250 µg/mL every 2–4 hours	250 µg/mL or 500 µg/2.5 mL	As prophylaxis of severe asthma or COPD	Slower onset of action, additive effect with salbutamol
Montelukast sodium; Montair, Ventair	10 mg OD for adults; 4–5 mg for children of 2–14 years	4 mg, 5 mg, 10 mg tab orally	Prophylaxis and treatment of chronic asthma, allergic rhinitis	Efficacy depends on the extent of mediator as leukotrienes
Sodium cromoglycate; Cromal, fintal	1–2 puffs 3–4 times/day or 1 rotacap/day	20 mg rotacap, inhaler, nasal spray	Prophylactic in mild to moderate asthma, allergic rhinitis	Useful only in long-term prophylaxis
Beclomethasone dipropionate; Beclate	100–200 µg BD titrated to 400 µg QID as inhalation	50 µg/100 µg/metered dose, 100 µg/200 µg rotacap	Mild to moderate asthma, perennial rhinitis	Should not exceed 600 µg/day to avoid systemic effects
Budesonide; Budecort, Pulmicort, Rhinocort	200–400 µg BD/TDS/QDS inhalation	100 µg/metered dose	Prophylaxis and treatment of asthma, allergic rhinitis	
Fluticasone propionate; Flohale, seroflo	100–250 µg BD, maximum 1000 µg/day	50, 100, 250 µg rotacap, inhaler, nasal spray	Mild, moderate and severe asthma	Longer duration, high potency

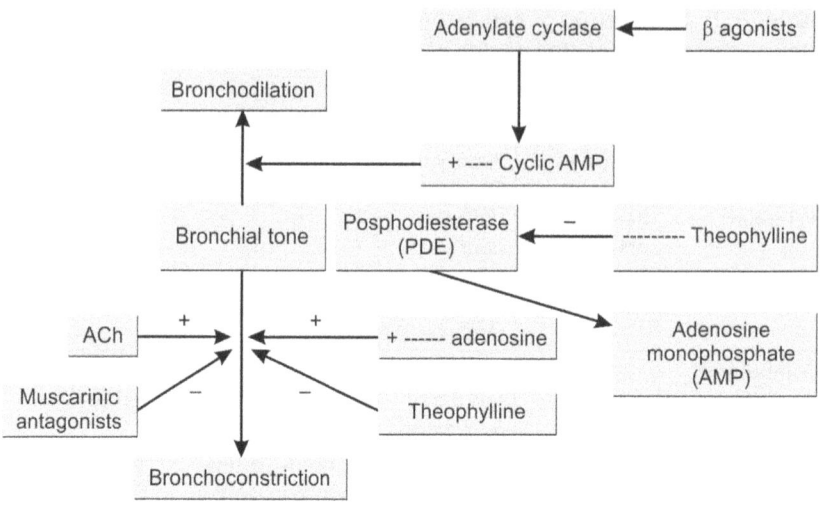

Fig. 13.1: Mechanism of action of bronchodilators.

   III. *Leukotriene antagonists*: Montelukast and zafirlukast.
   IV. *Mast cell stabilizers*: Na-cromoglycate, nedocromil sodium and ketotifen.
   V. *K^+ channel openers*: Cromakalim, levocromakalim, bimakalin, etc.

Others: NO donors mediator antagonists, e.g. kinin receptor antagonist—icatibant, H_1 receptor blockers, ketotifen, isoenzyme-selective PDE (III, IV) inhibitor piclamilast, anti-IgE Ab omalizumab, anti-asthma vaccine, novel corticosteroid ciclesonide and magnesium sulfate also have bronchodilator property.

SYMPATHOMIMETICS

These are the drugs mostly used for the management of asthma and are used as 'relievers'. Inhaled β_2 agonists are bronchodilator of choice in asthma. Non-selective β_2 agonists are only used as a last resort.

- *Mechanism*: Direct relaxation of the airway smooth muscle cells by stimulating adenylyl cyclase and increase in formation of cAMP in mast cells and other inflammatory cells and decrease in mediator release. The β_2 receptor on inflammatory cells are more prone to desensitization.
- β_2 *effect*: Relaxes smooth muscles of airway, inhibits mediator release and tachycardia and tremor (toxic effects).
- Presynaptic β_2 receptor inhibition may decrease in neurotransmission reducing reflex cholinergic bronchoconstriction.
- Precautions to be taken in the following: Hypertension, heart patients, those receiving digitalis.
- *Modes of administration*: Locally as aerosol or systemic.
- Aerosol therapy has better therapeutic ratio and minimal side effect.
- Inhaled β_2 agonists with short duration of action are preferred.

Aerosol Therapy

- Critical determination of the delivery of any particulate matter to the lungs is the size of the particles.
- 10 μm particles get deposited in the mouth, 0.5 μm in the alveoli, while 1-5 μm is the most effective particle size to reach the airway.
- Deep breath for 5-10 seconds followed by slow deep breathing is recommended.
- To minimize side effect, greater volume should be inhaled and swallowed drug should be kept to a minimum. Swallowed drug should have minimum absorption and high first pass metabolism. So use of large volume spacer is advised.

Types of Inhalers Used

1. *Pressurized metered dose inhalers*: Cheap and portable, large volume of spacer is attached.
2. *Nebulizers*: Administered by face mask. Suitable for elderly and children.
3. *Dry powder inhalers*: Require high airflow rate; dry powder may be irritating and requires proper storage.

Drugs

β_2-Selective Agonists (Flowchart 13.1)

Most effective bronchodilators. Oral dose is generally higher than inhaled dose leading to systemic adverse effects; should be used in patients unable to use inhalers. The IV route should be preserved for acutely ill patients.

Short-acting: Used for acute exacerbation as rescue medication, e.g. salbutamol, terbutaline, albuterol. Duration 1-5 minutes to 2-6 hours. Short-acting β_2 agonists like albuterol can be used as required for acute symptom relief. Oral slow release formulations are used occasionally as in nocturnal asthma.

Long-acting: Long side chain makes them more lipophilic, hence of long duration. Duration 4-8 hours, e.g. bambuterol, salmeterol, formoterol. Development of tolerance is common.

Side Effect of Inhalation
- Increase in heart rate, cardiac arrhythmias and CNS effects.

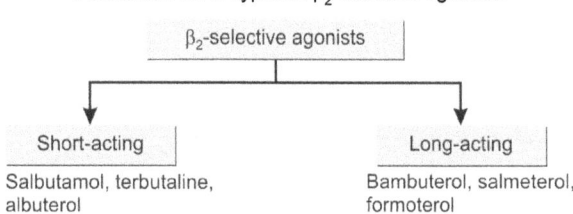

Flowchart 13.1: Types of β_2-selective agonists.

- *Systemic*: Tremor, muscle cramps, cardiac tachyarrhythmias, metabolic disturbances, e.g. increase in free fatty acid, glucose, lactate, hypokalemia and tolerance.
- *Salbutamol, terbutaline*: Inhalational therapy is mostly used to abort acute attacks. Onset is 5 minutes, duration 2–4 hours.
- *Bambuterol*: Prodrug of terbutaline, slowly hydrolized in plasma and lungs by pseudocholinesterase to release the active drug over 24 hours.
- *Salmeterol*: First long-acting selective β_2 agonist with a slow onset of action.
- *Formoterol*: Faster onset of action, i.e. 10 minutes and acts for 12 hours when inhaled.
  Epinephrine, ephedrine and isoprenaline are now rarely prescribed due to troublesome adverse effects, e.g. tachycardia, arrhythmias, worsening of angina pectoris. Long-acting agonists are useful for long-term control of asthma and chronic obstructive pulmonary disease (COPD).

METHYLXANTHINES

Methylxanthines like theophylline and caffeine have been in use since 1930s.

Methylated Xanthine Alkaloids

The three important methylxanthines are theophylline, theobromine and caffeine. Their major source is beverages (tea, coffee, and cocoa respectively). Though importance of theophylline in the treatment of asthma has waned, its low cost is an important advantage in economically disadvantaged patients.

A theophylline preparation commonly used for therapeutic purposes is aminophylline. A theophylline–ethylenediamine complex, enprofylline, a 3-propyl derivative and have potent bronchodilator action with minimum toxic effect. Doxofylline too has less side effect.

Mechanism

Inhibit several members of the phosphodiesterase enzyme family. Inhibition results in higher concentration of intracellular cyclic adenosine monophosphate (AMP) and in some tissues cyclic guanosine monophosphate (GMP). Hence, it relaxes smooth muscles of airway. Decrease in release of mediators from inflammatory cells.

Another proposed mechanism of action is inhibition of cell surface receptors for adenosine. Adenosine causes contraction of airway smooth muscles and provokes histamine release from mast cells.

Effects

They have effects on CNS, kidney, cardiac, skeletal and smooth muscles. Of the three, theophylline is most selective in its smooth muscle effects while caffeine has most marked CNS effects.
- *CNS effects*: Increase in cortical arousal, increase in alertness and loss of fatigue.

- *Side effect*: Nervousness, tremor.
- *Toxicity*: Medullary stimulation and convulsions.
- *CVS effects*: Positive chronotropic, positive inotropic, increase CO, relaxation of vascular and smooth muscles, except cerebral blood vessels. Peripheral resistance and blood pressure may slightly increase due to stimulation of vasomotor center and increase in blood viscosity may improve blood flow. (Pentoxifylline is used in treatment of intermittent claudication).
- *GIT effects*: Stimulate secretion of both gastric and digestive enzymes, increase in acid secretion.
- *Kidney effects*: Weak diuretic, increase in GFR, decrease in tubular reabsorption.
- *Effects on smooth muscles*: Bronchodilation, tolerance does not develop, inhibits Ag-induced release of histamine from lung tissue. Induces apoptosis of eosinophils and neutrophils.
- *Effects on skeletal muscles*: Improves contractility and reverses fatigue of the diaphragm in COPD patients.

Pharmacokinetics

- Well absorbed from GIT.
- Narrow therapeutic window (5-15 mg/L). Unwanted effects occur with plasma concentration >15 mg/L; >40 mg/L causes seizures, arrhythmias leading to death. It is metabolized by liver. Children clear theophylline faster than adults but neonates and young infants have slowest clearance. It requires measurement of plasma level during the therapy.
  Plasma concentration of theophylline with effects:
  - 35 mg/mL → Convulsion, shock, arrhythmia
  - 30 mg/mL → Delirium, worsening CV functions and extrasystole
  - 25 mg/mL → Agitation, tachypnea, flushing and hypotension
  - 20 mg/mL → Restlessness, tremor, vomiting and palpitation
  - 15 mg/mL → Nausea, headache, nervousness and insomnia
  - 10 mg/mL → Minimum side effect
- *Most common side effect*: Nausea, vomiting, headache and abdominal discomfort.

Factors Affecting Theophylline Clearance

- *Conditions where plasma t½ of theophylline increases*:
  - Cirrhosis of liver, CCF, acute pulmonary edema, cor pulmonale, acute viral diseases.
  - Drugs: Cimetidine, erythromycin, ciprofloxacin, allopurinol, oral contraceptives and caffeine.
- *Conditions where plasma t½ of theophylline decreases*:
  - In heavy smokers
  - Drugs: Alcohol, phenobarbitone, phenytoin, carbamazepine and rifampicin.

ANTICHOLINERGICS

- Inhalational mode of administration is preferred. Ipratropium and tiotropium are commonly used.
- *Mechanism*: It blocks cholinergic constrictor tone, acts primarily in larger airways.
- *Disadvantage*: Slow onset of action and lower potency compared to other bronchodilators.
- *Use*: Prophylactic use or in addition to salbutamol, to decrease its dose. It is more useful in chronic obstructive pulmonary disease (COPD) than acute asthma.
  The selective antimuscarinic agents by inhalational route are preferred and have minimum adverse effects. It is used for long-term treatment especially in COPD. Ipratropium and tiotropium do not affect mucociliary clearance. Only side effect is bitter taste. Glaucoma, urinary retention may be precipitated in elderly.

GLUCOCORTICOIDS

These are 21-C compounds having a cyclopentanoperhydrophenanthrene nucleus; one of the most useful groups of drugs used in the treatment of bronchial asthma. They do not cause bronchodilation but inhibit the late inflammatory phase and decrease the bronchial hyper-reactivity.

Mechanism of Action

Corticosteroids penetrate cells and bind to high affinity cytoplasmic receptor protein. Structural change occurs in steroid-receptor complex, and it allows its migration into the nucleus, also it binds to specific sites on the chromatin. Transcription of specific mRNA leading to regulation of protein synthesis. This process takes 30-60 minutes, so effects of corticosteroids are not immediate. Once the proteins are synthesized, effects persist than steroids itself, by widespread effects on gene transcription and benefits in asthma. It inhibits production of inflammatory cytokines, suppresses bronchial reactivity and bronchial mucus secretion. Also, it inhibits activation of inflammatory cells, macrophages, mast cells, T-lymphocytes, eosinophil, influence airway remodeling retarding the disease progression. Asthmatic patients who require β_2 agonists four or more times weekly are viewed as candidates for inhaled glucocorticoids.

Modes of Therapy

- *Oral or parenteral glucocorticoids* are effective in short-term therapy in patients not improving with bronchodilators alone. Hydrocortisone (3-4 mg/kg 8 hourly) or methyl prednisolone (1 mg/kg 8 hourly) parenterally or prednisolone 30-60 mg/day, may be given for 5-7 days and tapered off gradually. Prolonged steroid therapy will lead to adrenal suppression. Systemic therapy required in acute severe exacerbations or chronic severe asthma or lung infection. Usually, large doses produce adrenal suppression. Hydrocortisone 3-4 mg/kg is given every 6 hours.

Prednisolone 30–40 mg is used orally, daily. Dose to be tapered over a week during withdrawal.

Side effects of systemic steroids: Stunted growth in children, weight gain, osteoporosis, cataract, hypertension, delayed puberty, hyperglycemia and peptic ulcer.

Signs of steroid withdrawal: Precipitation of asthma, muscular pain, lassitude, depression and hypotension.

- *Aerosol or inhalational steroids*: Inhalational method is generally used. These are lipid-soluble, effective by aerosol and produce minimum systemic effects. These are beclomethasone, betamethasone, triamcinolone, budesonide, fluticasone, flunisolide. Usually given 2 puffs 4 times a day or 4 puffs twice daily. Systemic toxicity occurs at doses more than 1600 mg/day. Mometasone can also be used. Newer drugs require 2 puffs BD/OD.

Side effects of inhalational steroids: Oropharyngeal candidiasis and dysphonia are caused. Prolonged use may cause mucosal damage and precipitate chest infections. Prevention can be done by rinsing the mouth and gargling after every use of aerosol. Improvement of pulmonary infection occurs in 2–4 weeks, treatment continued for 10–12 weeks, then tapered off gradually. Thus steroids offer much more complete and sustained symptomatic relief than any other drug available.

MAST CELL STABILIZERS

Cromolyn Sodium and Nedocromil Sodium

These inhibit effectively both antigen-induced and exercise-induced asthma; chronic use slightly decreases overall level of bronchial reactions. It is insoluble in water and not absorbed orally; it is given by inhalation, 20 mg is given by aerosol 3 or 4 times a day. Effect is manifested after 4 weeks or more. It is effective only prophylactically.

Mechanism

Inhibits degranulation of sensitized mast cells on exposure to specific antigen thereby prevents release of inflammatory mediators. These are probably the safest drugs with no major side effects and can be used for prolonged periods.

Side effects: Throat irritation, cough, dryness of mouth, chest tightness.

LEUKOTRIENE PATHWAY INHIBITORS

Arachidonic acid → 5HPETE → LTA_4 → LTC_4 → LTD_4 → LTE_4

$\underbrace{\hspace{4cm}}_{\text{Cysteine leukotrienes}}$

5-lipoxygenase Inhibitors (Flowchart 13.2)

Zileuton and Genleuton: These prevent allergen, exercise or aspirin-induced asthma; decrease the dose of bronchodilators and are additive to inhaled glucocorticoids. Half-life of zileuton is 2.5 hours.

Flowchart 13.2: Pathway of leukotriene inhibitors.

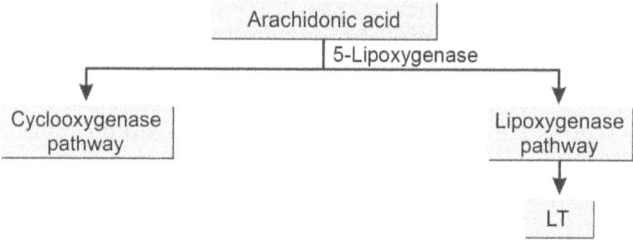

Short duration of action and hepatotoxic potential of 5 LO (lipoxygenase) inhibitors limit the use of 5 LO inhibitors.

Leukotriene Receptor Antagonists (Cys-LT$_1$ Receptor)

Montelukast, Pranlukast, and Zafirlukast: Used as add-on therapy of mild to moderate asthma. No role in acute severe attacks. These are administered orally once or twice daily. Good oral absorption, highly protein bound, metabolized in liver.

Side effects: Headache, rashes, Churg–Strauss syndrome (vasculitis of heart, kidney) half-life of 4–6 hours. Montelukast—Dose 10 mg in adults, 5 mg in children orally OD.

Ca Channel Blockers

Nifedipine, verapamil, nimodipine, nitrendipine, etc. inhibit allergen, exercise or antigen-induced asthma.

K⁺ CHANNEL OPENERS

Cromakalim, levocromakalim, bimakalin.
Review treatment every 1–6 months and gradually decrease the treatment.

Omalizumab

Humanized monoclonal antibody which prevents the binding of IgE to IgE receptors on mast cells. Also prevents binding of IgE to other inflammatory cells, e.g. macrophages, eosinophils. Used in severe asthma as SC injection every 2–4 weeks.
- *Others*: Ketotifen – 5HT and H$_1$ receptor antagonist also antagonizes PAF effects.
  It is orally active, inhibits release of histamine from mast cells. It decreases the number of attacks, severity and duration of acute attacks of asthma.
- *Side effect*: Sedation.
- *Azelastine*: Potent-inhibitor of smooth muscle contraction by histamine, ACh, 5 HT and LTC$_4$. Given orally in allergen or exercise-induced asthma.

TREATMENT OF STATUS ASTHMATICUS/ ACUTE SEVERE ASTHMA

Condition when severe attack has continued for more than 24 hours and the patient is not responding to the conventional therapy, is cyanosed, exhausted, dehydrated with pulse 120/min. Patient should be hospitalized immediately for treatment.

- Nebulized salbutamol and ipratropium bromide inhalation intermittently.
- Hydrocortisone 100 mg IV stat, then 100 mg 8 hourly.
- Humidified O_2 inhalation intermittently.
- Salbutamol/terbutaline 4 mg IM/SC to be given; as inhalational salbutamol may not be effective to reach through narrow bronchi.
- Correct dehydration and acidosis with saline and sodium bicarbonate/lactate infusion.
- Aminophylline 250–500 mg as 5% solution in 20 mL glucose given slowly IV in 15–20 min.
- Treat chest infection with intensive antibiotic therapy.

CHAPTER 14

Drugs Used in Cough

INTRODUCTION

Cough is a protective reflex and its purpose is to expel any respiratory secretions or foreign body from the air passages. It occurs due to—stimulation of mechano- or chemoreceptors in throat and air passages, stimulation of stretch receptors in the lungs.

Cough center is located in the upper part of the medulla. Stimulation of mechanoreceptors or chemoreceptors from tracheobronchial tree or lungs is carried via the glossopharyngeal and vagus nerves as efferent impulses to the cough center. The efferent impulses are carried via the parasympathetic and motor nerves to the diaphragm, intercostal muscles and the lung.

Cough may be productive or nonproductive. Productive cough is useful because it helps to expel the mucus and secretions of the airway tract but nonproductive cough fulfills no such purpose and is useless. Drugs for cough are classified in Flowchart 14.1.

Pharyngeal Demulcents: Cough lozenges, cough drops, linctuses, glycerin, liquorice.

Expectorants/Mucokinetics: Na/K citrate or acetate, potassium iodide, guaiacol/guaifenesin, tolu, balsam and ammonium salts.

Mucolytics: Bromhexine, acetylcysteine and carbocisteine.

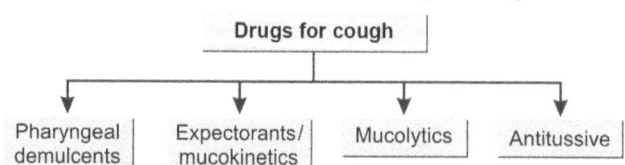

Flowchart 14.1: Classification of drugs for cough.

Antitussive
- *Opioids*: Morphine, codeine, pholcodine and noscapine.
- *Nonopioids*: Dextromethorphan, oxeladin and chlophedianol.
- *Antihistamines*: Chlorpheniramine, diphenhydramine and promethazine.

PHARYNGEAL DEMULCENTS

They soothe the throat directly as well as by promoting salivation and reduce afferent impulses from the inflamed/irritated pharyngeal mucosa.

EXPECTORANTS/MUCOKINETICS

- These increase the bronchial secretion or reduce the viscosity, facilitating its removal by coughing. Sodium and potassium citrate or acetate increases bronchial secretion by salt action. Potassium iodide secreted by bronchial glands and thereby increase in volume of secretion by irritant action. Contraindicated in acute bronchitis; also a gastric irritant, may induce hypothyroidism or goiter, also contraindicated in pregnant and nursing mothers.
- Guaiacol and its derivative guaiphenesin are synthetically prepared from wood or cresolite. Increase in bronchial secretion and mucociliary action, also gastric upset and rash can occur.
- *Others*: Ammonium chloride, syrup ipecac, volatile oils (eucalyptus, turpentine, camphor, thymol, menthol, etc.).

MUCOLYTICS

These help in expectoration by liquefying the viscous tracheobronchial secretions. Bromhexine is synthetic derivative of vasicine, an alkaloid from adhatoda vasica. It depolymerizes mucopolysaccharides directly as well as by liberating lysosomal enzymes, thus thinning thick, tenacious sputum; side effect rhinorrhea, lacrimation, gastric irritation and hypersensitivity. Ambroxol is a metabolite of bromhexine and is similar in action, side effect as bromhexine. Acetylcysteine opens the disulfide bonds in mucoproteins and makes it less acidic. It may be used as aerosol in patients of cystic fibrosis. Side effects are nausea, vomiting that may induce bronchospasm so contraindicated in asthma. Carbocisteine with its action similar to acetylcysteine. Contraindicated in peptic ulcer and first trimester of pregnancy.

ANTITUSSIVES

These act at CNS, to raise the threshold of cough and also peripherally decrease the tussal responses in the respiratory tract. These should only be used in:
- Dry, unproductive and irritating cough.
- Postoperative cases of abdominal operation, hernia, piles and cardiac patients.
- After ocular surgery.

Opiates

These are opium alkaloids, of which codeine has more selective action for cough center and treated as a standard antitussive.

- *Codeine*: Opium alkaloid, phenanthrine group, qualitatively similar to but less potent than morphine. It suppresses cough for about 6 hours. Abuse liability is low, constipation is the main side effect. In higher doses may cause respiratory depression, contraindication in asthmatics and patients with low respiratory drive.

Pholcodeine

No analgesic or addicting property; similar in efficacy to codeine but longer-acting.

Noscapine

Opium alkaloid of benzoisoquinoline series. It depresses cough but has no narcotic, analgesic or abuse liability. Side effects—headache, nausea, bronchospasm.

Nonopioids

Synthetic compounds having centrally acting antitussive property.

Dextromethorphan

The d-isomer has selective antitussive action. Effective as codeine but devoid of constipation and abuse liability. Side effects—dizziness, nausea, drowsiness, ataxia.

Oxeladin

Synthetic, centrally acting antitussive devoid of opioid side effect.

Chlophedianol

Similar to oxeladin, but has a slow onset of action and of longer duration. Others include carbetapentane, levopropoxyphene, benzonatate.

Antihistamines

H_1 antihistaminics afford relief in cough due to their sedative and anticholinergic actions, but lack selectivity for the cough center. They have no expectorant action, may even decrease by anticholinergic action. They are specially used for cough in respiratory allergic states.

Drugs for Dyspnea

- Bronchodilators relieve breathlessness due to airway obstruction.
- Chronic oxygen therapy is of benefit.
- Nebulized morphine may be of benefit in COPD.
- Nebulized furosemide reduces dyspnea of various etiology.

CHAPTER 15

Drugs Acting in Cardiovascular System

PATHOPHYSIOLOGY OF SHOCK AND ITS MANAGEMENT

Shock is a complex acute cardiovascular syndrome that results in a critical reduction in perfusion of vital tissues and a wide range of systemic effects. Shock is usually associated with hypotension, an altered mental state, oliguria and metabolic acidosis. If untreated, shock usually progresses to a refractory, deteriorating state and death.

The three major mechanisms responsible for shock are—
(i) Hypovolemia, (ii) cardiac insufficiency and (iii) altered vascular resistance.

Volume replacement and treatment of the underlying cause are the mainstays of the treatment of shock.

TYPES OF SHOCK

- Hypovolemic—due to acute loss of blood volume as in hemorrhage, acute diarrhea and vomiting.
  - Mechanism—reduced blood volume, → reduced preload, → reduced end-diastolic volume (EDV) → reduced cardiac output (CO).
- Cardiogenic shock—due to depression of cardiac contractility as in acute myocardial infarction (AMI), cardiomyopathy.
  - Decreased systolic blood pressure (BP) → increased LV filling pressure → pulmonary edema.
- Septic shock—endotoxins or bacterial wall lipopolysaccharides (LPS) released in gram-negative bacterial infection activate the immune system causing release of cytokines and inflammatory mediators.
  Lipopolysaccharides (LPS) → cytokine cascade → systemic vasodilation, resulting in decrease CO and decrease end-diastolic volume (EDV) due to widespread endothelial injury and liberation of nitric oxide (NO).
- Anaphylactic shock—due to acute anaphylaxis caused by allergen.
  Allergen → induce inflammatory mediators → systemic vasodilation → decrease CO.

- Neurogenic shock—neurogenic stimuli, which come into play are; → Depression of vasomotor center → decrease in CO.
It occurs due to—(i) high cervical cord injury, (ii) severe head injury, and (iii) cephalad migration of spinal anesthesia.

COMPENSATORY MECHANISMS

- Increased sympathetic discharge.
- Activation of renin-angiotensin system.
- Increased ACTH, increased aldosterone and increased ADH.
- Intense peripheral vasoconstriction, tachycardia.
- Hypoxia at cellular level → anaerobic metabolism → acidosis.

All these compensatory mechanisms further deteriorate the clinical condition ultimately leading to multiple end-organ damage and death.

So pharmacotherapy should be initiated as early as possible.

TREATMENT

General Measures

Initial therapy is aimed at maintaining systemic and coronary perfusion by raising systolic BP to more than 90 mm Hg and adjusting volume status to optimum LV filling pressure (PCWP—20 mm Hg)

Fluid Therapy

Blood loss should be replaced by blood. However, homologous blood is not always needed. Plasma substitute of choice should have—(a) an intravascular half-life of between 3 and 6 hours and (b) should be isotonic with plasma.

Various crystalloid solutions and colloid solutions have been employed to achieve normovolemic hemodilution. These are:

Ringer's lactate	Hydroxyethyl starch
5% albumin	Gelatin
Dextran	Combination of these agents

Polygeline solution has been described as an adequate plasma substitute. It has many desirable properties of an ideal agent and has an ideal half-life of about 4 hours.

Properties of an Ideal Plasma Replacement Fluid

- Oncotic pressure, pH and viscosity comparable with plasma.
- Optimal volume effect for a clinically adequate length of time.
- Improves microcirculation.
- Contains electrolytes, in particular calcium, in a similar concentration as in plasma.
- Restores or improves the renal function.
- Long shelf-life at extremes of temperature.
- Does not accumulate in tissues and cells.
- No dosage limitation.
- Does not overload the cardiovascular system.

- Does not cause edema formation.
- Noninterference with hemostasis.
- Does not interfere with or prevent a subsequent blood transfusion.

Ionotropes

Ionotropes increase cardiac contractility. A successful outcome in shock depends upon normalization of physiological function, which in turn depends on the reestablishment of adequate tissue O_2 delivery; which correlates to central venous pressure (CVP), mean arterial pressure (MAP), urine output and core-toe temperature.

Ionotropes change the contractility of myocardium. Ionotropic agents are a crucial component of the management strategy and the ultimate objective is to optimize tissue O_2 delivery.

Drugs used can be classified as—
- Catecholamines (Flowchart 15.1).
- Phosphodiesterase inhibitors.
- Digitalis glycosides.

The actions of catecholamines in critical condition differs from those seen in physiologically normal. Effect of contractility reduces due to subnormal number and function of β adrenoceptors. Activity of α receptors is decreased in septic shock. Types of catecholamine are shown in Flowchart 15.1.

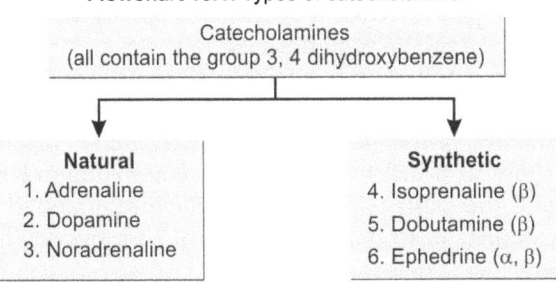

Flowchart 15.1: Types of catecholamine.

Sympathomimetics

Sympathomimetics are characterized in Table 15.1.

Table 15.1: Characteristics of sympathomimetics.

	$α_1$	$β_1$	$β_2$	DA	PDE
Noradrenaline	++	+			
Adrenaline	++	++	+		
Dopamine	++	++	+	++	
Dobutamine	+	++	++		
Dopexamine		+	++	+	
Milrinone					++

- *Adrenaline*: Causes increased stroke volume, increased CO, increased systolic blood pressure (BP), increased systemic vascular resistance (SVR), increased mean arterial pressure (MAP), bronchodilation, inhibits mast cell degranulation.
  Use—
  - In cardiac arrest in 1 in 10000 dilution in a dose of 10 mL slowly IV.
  - Anaphylactic shock—0.5 mL of 1 in 1000 dilution IM may be repeated every 5 minutes.
  - May be used in septic shock and cardiogenic shock when other sympathomimetics fail.
- *Noradrenaline*: Increased systemic vascular resistance (SVR), increased MAP, without significantly affecting cardiac output; improvement in renal function and urine output, can be given in septic shock.
- *Dopamine*: Direct action is dose related, dose is 2–5 µg/kg/min; Increased splanchnic and renal blood flow, increase in contractility of heart without affecting heart rate, hence lesser myocardial O_2 consumption.
- *Dopexamine*: Weak β_1 action, no α action. Its dopaminergic activity may increase renal perfusion, diuresis, natriuresis, can be used in septic shock.
- *Dobutamine*: Mixture of 2 isomers, produces dose dependent β_1 effect (predominant) with weak β_2 stimulation; positive ionotropic with minimal chronotropic action, MAP does not effect much, improves O_2 supply demand ratio of myocardium. Increases pulmonary shunt by perfusing unventilated alveoli, effective in cardiogenic shock and; all low flow states becomes less effective on prolonged use.
- *Isoprenaline*: Potent β_1, and β_2 agonistic action, β_2 effect is predominant in skin and muscles. Increase in heart rate, contractility, automaticity but potent dysrhythmogenic, causes peripheral vasodilation. Not useful in shock as it distributes blood to skin and muscles, increase in myocardial O_2 demand, used in management of profound bradycardia, specially complete heart block, treatment of Torsades de Pointes; also in cardiogenic shock; causes bronchodilation.

Phosphodiesterase Inhibitors

- *Amrinone*: Used IV.
- *Milrinone*: More potent. Inhibits phosphodiesterase (PDE) by increasing intracellular cyclic AMP and calcium. Causes decreased reuptake of calcium by sarcoplasmic reticulum, decreased peripheral, pulmonary, coronary resistance. Also causes increase in stroke volume, heart rate, cardiac output (CO) but mean arterial pressure (MAP) is unchanged, Used in treatment of cardiogenic shock, septic shock refractory to catecholamines.

Digitalis

Positive ionotropic effect, used in tachyarrhythmias.

Treatment of Anaphylactic Shock

- Adrenaline 0.5 mg. (0.5 mL of 1 in 1000 solution) IM repeat every 5-10 minutes.
- H_1 antihistaminic (chlorpheniramine 10-20 mg).
- IV glucocorticoid (hydrocortisone sodium succinate 100-200 mg) should be added in severe, recurrent cases. It acts slowly.

Treatment of Septic Shock

Antibiotics + hydrocortisone.

VASODILATORS

- Primarily causing decrease in preload → Glyceryl trinitrate, isosorbide dinitrate.
- Primarily causing decrease in afterload → Hydralazine, minoxidil, Ca^{+2} channel blocker (nifedipine), K^+ channel opener (nicorandil).
- Mixed/decrease in both preload and afterload→ACE inhibitors, AT_1 receptor antagonists/ARBs, α_1 blocker—prazosin, PDE inhibitors (amrinone milrinone) and nitroprusside.

SODIUM NITROPRUSSIDE (TABLE 15.2)

Uses

Its primary use is—
- To produce controlled hypotension.
- To control acute hypertensive crisis.
- To treat refractory cardiac failure specially after myocardial infarction.

Action

It relaxes both the resistance and capacitance and reduces total peripheral resistance as well as increases cardiac output by reducing afterload. Myocardial work is reduced, and there is decrease in preload and afterload. Ischemia is not accentuated and it improves ventricular function and CO in congestive heart failure (CHF) and ventricular dilatation.

Table 15.2: Comparative study of commonly used vasodilators.

Drug; (Generic and trade name)	Dose	Dosage form	Indications	Remarks
Sodium nitroprusside: (Nipride, Sonide)	0.5–6 µg/kg/min IV infusion	50 mg dissolved in 1 liter 5% dextrose	Hypertension, increased intracranial tension	Toxic if used in high dose and for prolonged period
Glyceryl trinitrate: (Angised, Nitrocontin)	0.4–0.8 mg sublingual/spray; 5–20 µg/min IV infusion	5–15 mg tab, spray, sublingual tablet, inj	Angina pectoris, hypertension, hypertensive emergency	Brief transient action, tolerance occurs after 18–24 hr of infusion
Hydralazine: (Zinepress, Nipresol)	0.1–0.5 mg/kg/dose IV 6–8 hrly	25–50 mg oral tablet	To lower BP in eclampsia	Contraindicated in aortic dissection, MI
Captopril: (Capotril, Angiopril)	25 mg BD to 50 mg TDS	12.5 mg, 25 mg tablet	To lower BP	Peak action occurs in 1 hr
Nifedipine: (Calcigard, Nifelat)	5–20 mg BD/TDS	5, 10, 20 mg tab	To lower BP	Reflex tachycardia

Mechanism of Action

- Endothelial cells, RBCs split nitroprusside to generate NO which relaxes vascular smooth muscle.
- Moreover nitroprusside is nonenzymatically converted to NO (and CN) by glutathione.

Dose

50 mg is added to a 500 mL bottle of 5% Dextrose solution. Infusion is started at 0.02 mg/min or 20-300 µg/min. Drug of choice in hypertensive crisis.

- *Side effect*: Due to vasodilatation, e.g. palpitation, nervousness, vomiting, perspiration, pain in abdomen, weakness, disorientation. Nitroprusside is split to release—cyanide (CN) which is converted to thiocyanate in liver; excess of thiocyanate may cause psychosis. It decomposes at alkaline pH or exposure to sunlight.
- *Drawbacks*: Need for careful continuous monitoring, light sensitivity, severe risk of cyanide toxicity.
- *Onset of action*: Starts within minutes, plasma half-life 7 days.
- (Nitroprusside → cyanmethemoglobin → free cyanide in RBC → thiocyanate in liver → cleared by kidneys).
- *Contraindication*: Systolic BP less than 90 mm Hg, diastolic less than 60 mm Hg, hepatic/renal failure.
- Precautions to be undertaken:
   a. Infusion at minimum dose, not longer than 10 minutes duration.
   b. Always shield it from light.
   c. Solution in normal saline and alkaline solution to be avoided.
   d. Discard if the solution is more than 4 hours old or discolored.

GLYCERYL TRINITRATE

- It is a volatile liquid which is adsorbed on the inert matrix of the tablet.
- It can be used sublingually or crushed under teeth.
- Onset of action within 1-2 minutes.
- Plasma ½ life—2 minutes.
- Cutaneous application as ointment/transdermal patch provides steady drug delivery; 4-6 hours and 24 hours, respectively.
- It acts sublingually within 5 minutes; duration 4-6 hours.
- IV infusion produces rapid steady plasma concentration; 5 µg/min titrated as needed.

Action

- It dilates veins more than arteries; preload reduction with peripheral pooling of blood. Decrease in venous return, decrease in end diastolic volume of heart, decrease in ventricular radius is observed.
- Some arteriolar dilatation, decrease in total peripheral resistance (TPR) or afterload on heart; decrease in BP, rate of decrease is systolic more than diastolic.

- Redistribution of coronary flow occurs. Nitrates preferentially relax bigger conducting coronary arteries than arterioles/resistance vessels. No direct stimulant or depressant action on heart.
- It tends to decongest lungs by shifting blood to systemic circulation. Bronchi, biliary tract and esophagus are relaxed.
- Dilate cutaneous and meningeal vessels causing flushing and headache.

Mechanism of Action

Release reactive free radical nitric oxide, with increase in cGMP, increase in dephosphorylation of myosin light chain kinase. It interferes with activation of myosin and fails to interact with actin to cause contraction.

Glyceryl trinitrate (GTN) and isosorbide dinitrate are short acting in sublingual route but of longer duration by oral route.

- *Side effect*: Throbbing headache, flushing, sweating, palpitation, tolerance, rarely methemoglobinemia and rashes.
- *Uses*: Angina pectoris, acute coronary syndrome, congestive heart failure (CHF) and left ventricular failure (LVF), myocardial infarction (MI), esophageal spasm and cyanide poisoning (sodium nitrite).

HYDRALAZINE

- It is a directly acting arteriolar vasodilator.
- Little action on venous capacitance vessels.
- Pharmacokinetics—well absorbed orally. It has low bioavailability (BA), high first-pass metabolism, plasma t½ = 1.5–3 hours. However, higher doses result in greater vasodilation, but chances of development of systemic lupus erythematosus (SLE).

Actions

Arteriolar dilatation with reduction in total peripheral resistance (TPR). There is greater reduction of diastolic BP than systolic. Reflex compensatory mechanism due to tachycardia, increase in CO and renin release leads to increase in aldosterone, increase in Na^+ and H_2O retention.

Mechanism of Action

It causes generation of endothelium dependent NO or decreases intracellular calcium concentration.

- *Pharmacokinetics*: It is well absorbed orally and undergoes first pass metabolism. BA is high in slow acetylators in whom SLE can develop.
- *Side effects*: Mainly due to vasodilation; flushing, headache, dizziness, palpitation, fluid retention, edema. Paresthesias, tremor, muscle cramp, peripheral neuritis, SLE or rheumatoid arthritis on prolonged use.
- Use:
    - As antihypertensive in moderate to severe hypertension.
    - It can be used in patients with renal involvement.
    - In treatment of hypertension during pregnancy.

MINOXIDIL

It is similar to hydralazine but it is a prodrug, active metabolite is an opener of ATP operated K^+ channels and is also used in alopecia.

VASODILATORS IN HEART FAILURE

In congestive heart failure (CHF), the impaired contractile function of the heart is exacerbated by compensatory increases in both preload and afterload. Preload is the volume of blood that fills the ventricle during diastole. Elevated preload causes over filling of the heart, which increases the workload. Afterload is the pressure that must be overcome for the heart to pump blood into the arterial system. Elevated afterload causes the heart to work harder and pump blood into the arterial system. Vasodilators are useful in reducing excessive preload and afterload.

Dilatation of venous blood vessels leads to a decrease in cardiac preload by increasing venous capacitance; arterial dilators reduce systemic arteriolar resistance and decrease afterload.

Vasodilators with differing profiles of arteriolar and venodilator action are available;
- Arteriolar dilators (primarily decrease afterload):
  - Hydralazine
  - Minoxidil
  - Ca^{+2} channel blockers
  - Potassium channel openers.
- Venodilators (primarily decrease preload)
  - Nitrates—GTN, isosorbide dinitrate, nitroglycerin.
- Mixed dilators (decrease in both preload and afterload)
  - ACE inhibitors, ARBs, prazosin, phentolamine, nitroprusside.
  - For symptomatic treatment of acute heart failure, choice of IV vasodilator depends on the primary hemodynamic abnormality in the individual patient. In the long-term survival, benefit has been obtained only with a combination of hydralazine and isosorbide dinitrate or with ACE inhibitors. In this case the latter performing better than the former. Drugs with both preload and afterload are most effective. Only ACE inhibitors and AT_1 antagonists losartan alter the course of pathological changes in CHF. They provide symptomatic as well as disease modifying benefits by retarding or reversing ventricular hypertrophy and remodeling. Prognostic benefits have been established in mild to severe CHF as well as in patients with asymptomatic systolic dysfunction. They are thus recommended for all grades of congestive heart failure (CHF), unless contraindicated or if renal function deteriorates.
  - Nitrovasodilators have long been used in the treatment of heart failure and remain among the most widely used vasoactive medications in clinical practice. These drugs relax vascular smooth muscle by supplying NO and thereby activating soluble guanylyl cyclase. Thus the

drugs mimic the actions of endogenous NO, an intracellular and paracrine autacoid formed by the conversion of arginine to citrulline by a family of enzymes termed NO synthases. These enzymes are widely distributed and are found in endothelial and smooth muscle cells throughout the vasculature.
- Sodium nitroprusside prodrug and potent vasodilator is effective in reducing both ventricular filling pressures and systemic vascular resistance. It has rapid onset and offset of action and dose can be titrated according to the desired hemodynamic effect. Combination of preload and afterload reduction improve myocardial energetics by reducing wall stress. Nitroprusside is particularly effective in patients with CHF due to elevations of systemic vascular resistance and or mechanical complications that follow acute myocardial infarction (AMI). Hypotension is a common adverse effect.
- IV nitroglycerin like nitroprusside is a vasoactive NO source that is commonly used in cardiac care units. In patients with CHF, IV nitroglycerine is most clearly indicated in the treatment of left heart failure due to acute myocardial infarction (AMI). Its use is limited by headache and development of nitrate tolerance.
- Organic nitrates are available in a number of formulations that include rapid acting tablets or sprays or topical application or ointments or patches. They are relatively safe agents whose principal action in treatment of congestive heart failure (CHF) is reduction in left ventiricular (LV) filling pressures, due to increase in peripheral venous capacitance. These drugs have a selective vasodilator effect on the epicardial coronary vasculature and may enhance both systolic and diastolic ventricular function by increasing coronary flow.
- The mechanism that underlies the vasodilator activity of hydralazine remain poorly understood. In heart failure, hydralazine reduces right and left ventricular afterload by decreasing pulmonary and systemic vascular resistance. This results in augmentation of forward stroke volume and a decrease in ventricular systolic wall stress. Hydralazine is effective in decreasing renal vascular resistance and in increasing renal blood flow to a greater degree than are most other vasodilators with the exception of ACE inhibitors. As hydralazine has minimal effects on venous capacitance and therefore is most effective when combined with agents with venodilating activity.
- Amplodipine and felodipine have less negative ionotropic effect compared to other calcium channel blockers and can be used cautiously to decrease sympathetic nervous activity. Minoxidil causes arteriolar dilatation but not capacitance vessels. It may cause severe reflex tachycardia which is deleterious for the already decompensated heart. Moreover it causes Na and water retention which will add to the burden of volume overload, hence contraindicated in congestive heart failure (CHF).

Newer Development

A synthetic form of the endogenous BNP recently approved in acute cardiac failure in nesiritide. This recombinant product increases cGMP in smooth muscle cells and effectively reduces venous and arteriolar tone and also causes diuresis. It has short plasma ½ life (18 minutes) and administered as a bolus IV dose followed by continuous infusion.

Bosentan, an orally active competitive inhibitor of endothelin is under clinical trial, has been approved for use in pulmonary hypertension.

β-BLOCKERS

β-blocking drugs occupy β-receptors and competitively reduce receptor occupancy by catecholamines and other β agonists. Most β-blockers in clinical use are pure antagonists while some are partial agonists. Partial agonists inhibit the activation of β-receptors in the presence of high catecholamine concentration but moderately activate the receptors in the absence of endogenous agonists.

CLASSIFICATION (FLOWCHARTS 15.2 AND 15.3)

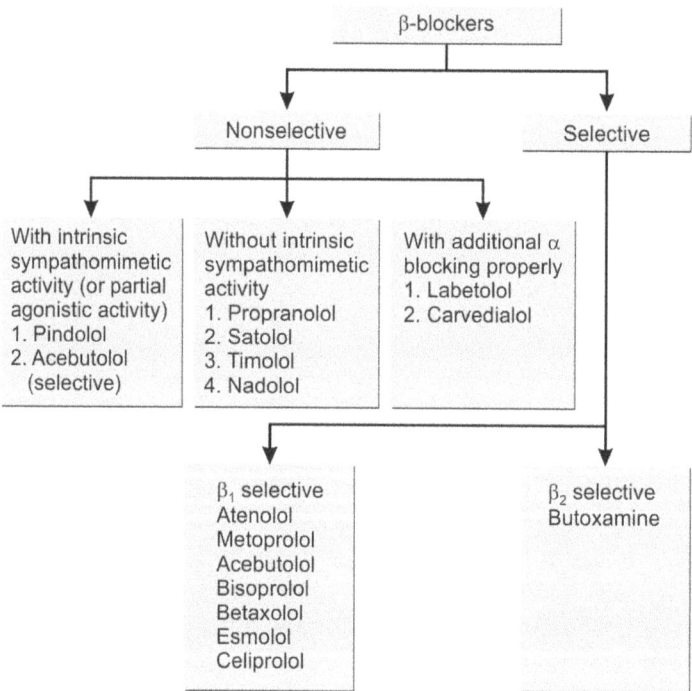

Flowchart 15.2: Selective and nonselective β-blockers.

Classification According to Pharmacological Properties and Time of Development

Chemically the β-receptor antagonist drugs resemble isoproterenol. A potent β-receptor antagonist propranolol is the prototype β antagonist. Other β-blockers differ in the following properties:
- Relative affinity for $β_1$ and $β_2$ receptors.
- Intrinsic sympathomimetic activity.
- Blockade of α receptors.
- Differences in lipid solubility.

Flowchart 15.3: First-, second-, and third-generation β-blockers.

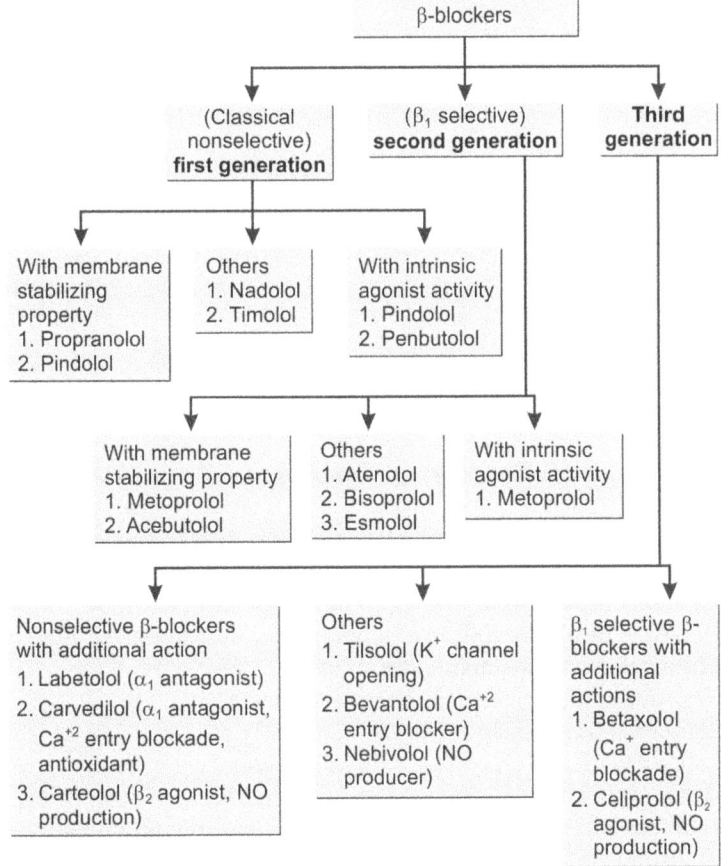

- Capacity to induce vasodilation.
- Pharmacokinetic properties.

PHARMACOKINETICS

- Most drugs are well absorbed after oral administration.
- Peak concentration in 1–3 hours.
- Bioavailability varies for most β antagonists with the exception of betaxolol, penbutolol, pindolol and satolol.
- Rapidly distributed.
- Large volume of distribution.
- Most β blockers have plasma ½ life of 3–10 hours except esmolol which has a plasma ½ life of 10 minutes, Nadolol has longest plasma ½ life.
- Propranolol and metoprolol are extensively metabolized in the liver, atenolol, celiprolol and pindolol are less completely metabolized, nadolol is excreted unchanged.

PHARMACODYNAMICS (FIG. 15.1)

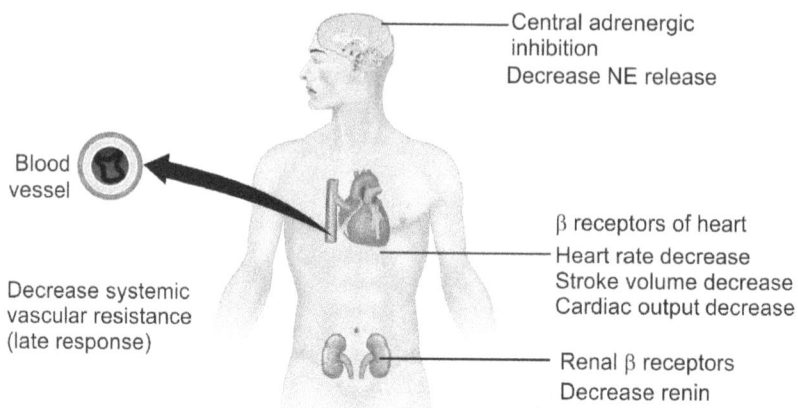

Figure 15.1: Actions of β-blockers.

- CVS-β-receptor blockade has relatively little effect on the normal heart of an individual at rest but has profound effects when sympathetic control of the heart is dominant.
    - Decrease in BP (inhibition of angiotensin-aldosterone system, central actions decrease sympathetic outflow).
    - Negative ionotropic and chronotropic effects.
    - $β_2$ mediated vasodilation.
    - Cardiac work and O_2 consumption decreases.
    - Decrease in automaticity and rate of ectopic foci.
    - Total peripheral resistance decreases on chronic administration due to chronically reduced CO.
- Respiratory tract
    - Bronchoconstriction, increasing airway resistance specially in patients with asthma.
- CNS – subtle behavioral changes.
    - Forgetfulness, increase in dreaming and nightmares.
    - Propranolol relieves anxiety due to peripheral rather than central action.
- Eye
    - Decrease in intraocular tension specially in glaucomatous eye.
    - Decrease in secretion of aqeous humor.
    - No consistent action on pupil size or accommodation.
- Metabolic and endocrine effects:
    - Inhibit lipolysis.
    - Glycogenolysis in liver is partially inhibited also in heart and skeletal muscle.
    - Plasma triglyceride level and LDL:HDL ratio is increased during propranolol therapy.
    - Prolonged therapy may cause carbohydrate intolerance due to decrease in insulin release.

- Effects not related to β-blockade:
  - Intrinsic sympathomimetic activity→prevents bronchoconstriction and bradycardia.
  - Local anesthetic/membrane stabilizing property.
  - Propranolol inhibits adrenergetically provoked tremor on muscle fiber.
- Uterus—relaxation.

USES OF β-BLOCKERS (TABLE 15.3)

- Hypertension.
- *Ischemic heart disease*: Propranolol, timolol or metoprolol can be used.
- *Cardiac arrhythmias*: Satolol and esmolol.
- *Myocardial infarction*: To decrease infarct size and minimize complications.
- *CHF*: Mild-to-moderate CHF to decrease myocyte apoptysis and remodeling.
- Dissecting aortic aneurysm.
- *Pheochromocytoma*: Administration after α-blockade to control tachycardia and arrhythmia.
- *Glaucoma*: Timolol, betaxolol, carteolol, levobunolol and betaxolol; decrease in aqeous formation and decrease in IOT.
- *Thyrotoxicosis*: It inhibits peripheral conversion of T_4 to T_3 and controls symptoms.
- *Migraine prophylaxis*: Decrease in frequency and intensity of migraine headache.
- *Anxiety*: It relieves symptoms.
- Essential tremor.
- Hypertropic obstructive cardiomyopathy.

ADVERSE EFFECTS

- *CVS*: It can precipitate CHF and edema, bradycardia specially in patients with sick sinus. β-blockers can interact with calcium channel antagonist, e.g. verapamil to cause hypotension, bradycardia, heart failure and other cardiac conduction anomalies.
- *Respiratory*: Worsening of preexisting asthma, or other forms of airway obstruction.
- *Worsens or exacerbates*: Prinzmetal's angina due to unopposed α mediated coronary constriction. Exacerbation of severe peripheral vascular disease/vasospastic disorders.
- Carbohydrate intolerance in prediabetics.
- Deleterious lipid profile, increase in LDL cholesterol, decrease in HDL level.
- *Sudden withdrawal of drug causes*: Rebound hypertension or exacerbation of angina due to upregulation of β-receptors.
- Tiredness and decrease in exercise capacity.
- *Contraindicated in insulin-dependent diabetes*: Symptoms of hypoglycemia are obliterated.

Table 15.3: Comparative study of some commonly used β-blockers.

Drug; (Generic and trade name)	Dose	Dosage	Indication	Remarks
Propranolol: (Inderal, Betabloc)	40–160 mg BD–QID	10, 40, 80 mg tab	Anxiety, tremor, arrhythmia	Nonselective β-blocker
Metoprolol: (Metolar, Betaloc)	100 mg OD/50 mg BD	12.5 SR, 25 mg, 50 mg tab	Preferred in diabetics on oral antidiabetics or insulin	5–15 mg inj may be given in MI
Atenolol; Aten, Betacard	50–100 mg OD	50, 100 mg tab	Most commonly used	Long-acting
Esmolol: (Miniblock)	0.5 mg/kg followed by 0.05–0.2 mg/kg	100 mg/10 mL amp, 250 mg/10 mL inj.	Intraoperative BP management	Ultra short. acting
Celiprolol: (Celipres)	200–600 mg OD	100, 200 mg tab	Hypertension and CHF in asthmatics	Mild β_2 agonistic action
Nebivolol: (Nebicard, Nodon)	2.5–5 mg OD	2.5 mg, 5 mg tablet	CHF, hypertension with hyperlipidemia, diabetes, Elderly	Beneficial on carbohydrate and lipid metabolism

- Contraindicated in partial and complete heart block as—cardiac arrest may occur.
- CNS: Sleep disturbance, forgetfulness and depression.

As abrupt withdrawal of β-blocker from chronic therapy, may lead to 'rebound hypertension', β-blockers should be tapered over 2 weeks.

β-BLOCKERS IN HEART FAILURE

The use of β-blockers in chronic heart failure—improves symptoms, reduces hospitalization, decrease mortality in mild and moderate heart failure.

Accordingly β-blockers are now recommended for routine use in patients with (a) ejection fraction less than 35%, (b) New York Heart Association (NYHA) class II or III symptoms; in combination with ACE inhibitor or angiotensin receptor antagonist and diuretics as required.

Suggested mechanisms of action of β-blockers—
- Attenuation of adverse effects of catecholamines (including apoptysis).
- Upregulation of β-receptors.
- Decrease in heart rate.
- Reduces remodeling due to inhibition of the mitogenic activity of catecholamines.
- Reduce oxidative stress in myocardium.

More recent data indicate that β-antagonist therapy may attenuate the hyperphosphorylation of the ryanodine (RyR) receptor that has been linked to abnormal intracellular Ca^{+2} handling in experimental models of heart failure.

Of the β-blockers, bisoprolol, carvedilol and metoprolol have shown to reduce mortality in various studies.

Since β-blockers have the potential to worsen both ventricular function and symptoms in patients with heart failure, the following points are to be maintained—
- It should be initiated at less than $1/10$th of final dose.
- Dose to be increased slowly over weeks under careful supervision.
- Increase in tendency to retain fluid will require adjustment in diuretic regimen.
- Class IIIB and IV heart failure patients should be approached with great caution.
- New onset heart failure patients should not be treated until they have stabilized for several days to weeks.

Point to note (evidence based): Perioperative beta blockade may reduce the risk of MI but may increase the risk of stroke and death.

INOTROPIC AGENTS AND VASOCONSTRICTORS

The comparative study of some ionotropic agents and vasoconstrictors are given in Table 15.4.

ADRENALINE

Prototype sympathomimetic stimulates both α and β receptors.

Actions

BP—potent vasopressor; Given IV, it produces typical response. Rise in BP with systolic rise > diastolic, so increase pulse pressure.

Mechanism

- Direct myocardial stimulation, increase heart rate, peripheral vasoconstriction.
- As response wanes, mean BP may fall below normal. Biphasic response to larger dose is due to increase sensitivity of adrenaline to vasodilator β_2 receptor than vasoconstrictor α receptors. Slow IV or SC infection does not produce such response.
- *Blood vessels*: Constriction of smaller arterioles and precapillary vessels. Blood flow to skeletal muscles are increased. Constriction predominates in cutaneous mucous membrane and renal beds.
- *Heart*: Powerful cardiac stimulant, directly stimulates myocardium and pacemaker cells. Heart rate increase, rhythm may be altered. Cardiac output increase, work of heart and O_2 consumption are markedly increased.
- *Respiratory system*: Relaxes bronchial muscle, decongests bronchial mucosa. Also inhibits Ag-induced release of inflammatory mediators.
- *GI system*: GI smooth muscles is relaxed. Intestinal tone and frequency of contraction decrease. Stomach is relaxed and pyloric, ileocecal sphincters are contracted.
- *Bladder*: Detrusor is relaxed; trigone is contracted; inhibits micturition.
- *Uterus*: Adrenaline contracts/relaxes in different species.
- *CNS*: In conventional therapeutic doses does not enter central nervous system (CNS). May cause restlessness, apprehension, headache and tremor.
- *Metabolic*: Increase Blood glucose, lactate and FFA.
  - *Dose*—0.2-0.5 mg SC, IM action lasts ½-2 hours.
  - Local vasoconstrictor : 1:200000
    1:100000
  - *Uses*—anaphylaxis, bronchial asthma, heart block, cardiac arrest, decongestant, with local anesthetics, in epistaxis, in eye for mydriasis, failure of heart.
  - Contraindicated in patients receiving nonselective β-blockers, coronary artery disease, moderate to severe hypertension.

NORADRENALINE

Sympathomimetic with agonistic action at α_1, α_2 and β_1 receptors. Similar potency as adrenaline but with little effect on β_2 receptors.

Actions

- Increase peripheral resistance and both diastolic and systolic BP increase.
- Positive ionotropic action on heart.
- Cardiac output is unchanged.
- Vagal reflex causes bradycardia.
- Decreased blood flow to organs, e.g. liver, kidney, mesenteric and splanchnic vessels.
- Coronary blood flow is usually increased.

Pharmacokinetics

- Not absorbed orally.
- Absorbed poorly when given SC.
- Metabolized by same enzymes as adrenaline.
- Metabolic products are found in urine.

Adverse Effects

- Severe hypertension.
- Sloughing may occur at the injection site.
- Reduced perfusion to organs like kidney, intestines may be a source of danger.

Uses

- Hypotension, shock.
- Dose = 2–4 µg/min. IV infusion.
- Available in 2 mg/2 mL amp.

DOPAMINE

- Immediate metabolic precursor of NE and epinephrine.
- As a central neurotransmitter it is important in regulation of movement.
- In the periphery it is synthesized in the epithelial cells of proximal tubules (PT) and is thought to extert local diuretic and natriuretic effects.

Actions

- At low concentration it interacts with vascular D_1 receptors specially in renal, mesenteric and coronary beds → Vasodilation.
- Low dose dopamine causes increase in GFR, renal blood flow (RBF) and Na^+ excretion.
- In moderate concentration it has positive ionotropic effect on myocardium due to action on β_1 receptors → tachycardia, increased systolic blood pressure (SBP), increased pulse pressure, diastolic BP and total peripheral resistance remain unchanged.

- At higher concentration, dopamine activates vascular α_1 receptors, leading to generalized vasoconstriction.
- Dopamine has no CNS effects as it cannot cross the blood-brain barrier (BBB).

Dose

0.2–1 mg/min IV; available as 200 mg. in 5 mL ompoule.

Adverse Effects

Tachycardia, arrhythmia, angina, hypertension, headache is common. Extravasation may cause sloughing of skin.

Uses

Severe CCF specially with oliguria, cardiogenic and septic shock.

DOBUTAMINE

- Structurally resembles dopamine but activity due to activation of α and β-receptors.
- Clinical preparation is a racemic mixture; at clinical dose it is a cardio-stimulant with relative selective action.
- Potent β_1-receptor agonist.
- It is more ionotropic than chronotropic.
- It enhances automaticity of the SA node.
- Total peripheral resistance is not greatly affected. CO increases and heart rate also increases.

Adverse Effects

Increases BP, tachycardia, atrial fibrillation or ventricular ectopic activity. Tolerance may develop after a few days.

Uses

- Short-term treatment of cardiac decompensation following cardiac surgery, myocardial infarction or CCF.
- Onset of effect is rapid, plasma t½ = 2 minutes; steady state of concentration is achieved in 10 minutes.
- Rate of infusion = 2.5–10 µg/kg/minutes. Available as 50 mg/4 mL in ampoule.

PHENYLEPHRINE

- Relatively pure α_1 agonist.
- Longer duration of action compared to the catecholamines.
- Effective mydriatic and decongestant.
- Activates β receptors only at high concentrations.
- Causes marked vasoconstriction (arterial) during IV infusion.
- Raises blood pressure (BP).

Uses

- To raise BP in hypotensive states.
- Nasal decongestant.
- Mydriatic.

MEPHENTERMINE

- Sympathomimetic drug that acts both directly on α and β receptors and indirectly, by releasing NA.
- Onset of action in 5-15 minutes after IM injection; effect lasts for several hours (2-6 hours).
- Increased cardiac contraction, increased CO, increased systolic and diastolic BP.
- Change in heart rate is variable.

Side Effect

CNS stimulation, excess increase in BP and arrhythmia.

Use

To raise BP during spinal anesthesia, cardiogenic shock, other hypotensive states.

METARAMINOL

Direct α receptor agonist; indirectly raises noradrenaline (NA) release.

Uses

Hypotensive state, paroxysmal arterial tachycardia when associated with hypotension.

MIDODRINE

- Orally effective $α_1$ receptor agonist.
- Prodrug, active metabolite is desglymidodrine.
- Duration of action 4-6 hours.

Uses

To treat postural hypotension, autonomic insufficiency.

Dose

2.5 mg-10 mg TDS thrice daily.

MILRINONE

- Ionotropic vasodilator.
- Phosphodiesterase -3 inhibitor.
- Should not be used for prolonged period, better less than 48 hours; otherwise chances of ventricular arrhythmia and mortality.

- Slow IV infusion over 10 minutes at 50 µg/kg followed by 0.50 µg kg/min for up to 12 hours.

Use
Short-term management of chronic heart failure.

Contraindications
Acute myocardial infarction (AMI), tight aortic stenosis; hypertrophic obstructive subaortic stenosis.

Table 15.4: Comparative study of some commonly used drugs as ionotropic agents and vasoconstrictors.

Drug; (Generic and trade name)	Dose	Dosage	Remarks
Adrenaline: (Adrenaline)	0.1 mL/kg/dose of 1:10,000 in cardiac arrest; 0.01 mL/kg of 1:1000 in anaphylaxis; 0.1–1 µg/kg/min infusion in shock	1 mg/mL of 1:1000 dilution inj	Administered slowly under close monitoring
Noradrenaline: (Nordrin, Norad, Adrenor)	2–4 µg/min IV infusion	2 mg/2 mL inj amp	Extravasation may cause local tissue necrosis
Dopamine: (Dopamine, Dopacard)	5 µg/kg/min; (1 mL in 100 mL 5% Dextrose = 400 µg/mL)	40 mg/mL inj, 200 mg in 5 mL amp.	Drip rate closely monitored to maintain renal perfusion
Dobutamine: (Dobustat, Dobutrex, Dobutam)	5–20 µg/kg/min IV infusion	50 mg/mL, 250 mg/ 5 mL vial	Used in shock unresponsive to fluid therapy, CCF
Digoxin: (Lanoxin, Digox)	40–50 µg/kg/day oral; 2/3rd dose parenteral; maintenance is 1/4th of oral dose	0.25 mg tab, 0.5 mg/2 mL inj	Refractory cases of heart failure
Amrinone: (Amicor)	0.75 mg/kg IV foll by 2–20 mg/kg/min	100 mg/20 mL	Ionotrope and vasodilator
Mephentermine: (Mephentin)	0.4 mg/kg/dose	15 mg/mL, 30 mg /10 mL, 10 mg tab	Used in hypotension

DRUGS USED IN HYPERTENSION

Hypertension is a clinical condition, when BP of an individual is beyond the limit of 140/90 mm Hg. British Hypertension Society suggests drugs are needed if sustained diastolic more than 100 mm Hg on ≥3 readings 1 week apart or sustained diastolic is more than 90 mm Hg over 6 months on several occasions or isolated systolic is more than 160 mm Hg or any end-organ damage. For diabetic patients or patients with renal disease with BP >130/80 mm Hg.

CAUSES

- 95% essential or unknown.
- *Renal*: Renal A stenosis, polycystic kidneys, chronic pyelonephritis and glomerulonephritis.
- *Endocrine*: Cushing's, Conn's syndrome, pheochromocytoma, acromegaly and hyperparathyroidism.
- *Others*: Coarctation of aorta, preeclampsia, prolonged steroid therapy.

In both normal and hypertensive individuals, cardiac output and peripheral resistance are controlled by two overlapping control mechanisms (Fig. 15.2).

- The baroreflexes mediated by the sympathetic nervous system.
- The renin angiotensin aldosterone system.

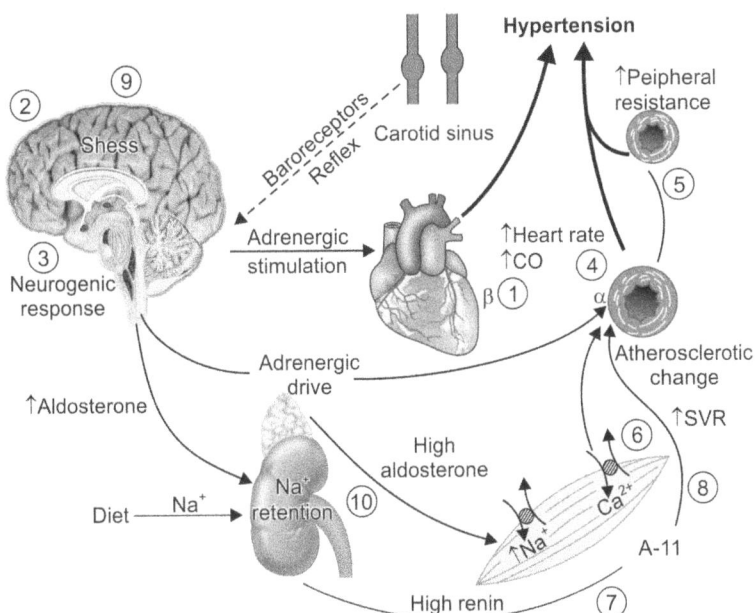

Figure 15.2: Sites of antihypertensive action.

(1) β-blockers: Atenolol acebutolol; (2) Centrally acting: Clonidine, methyldopa; (3) Post-ganglionic sympathetic nerve terminal blocker—guanethidine; (4) α$_1$-receptor blocker: Prazosin, terazosin; (5) Vasodilators: Minoxidil, nitroprusside, hydralazine; (6) Calcium channel blockers: Amlodipine felodipine; (7) ACE-inhibitors: Enalapril, lisinopril; (8) Angiotensin receptor blockers: Losartan, telmisartan; (9) New generation centrally acting: Moxonidine; (10) Diuretics: Hydrochlorothiazide, indapamide

Flowchart 15.4: Factors influencing blood pressure.

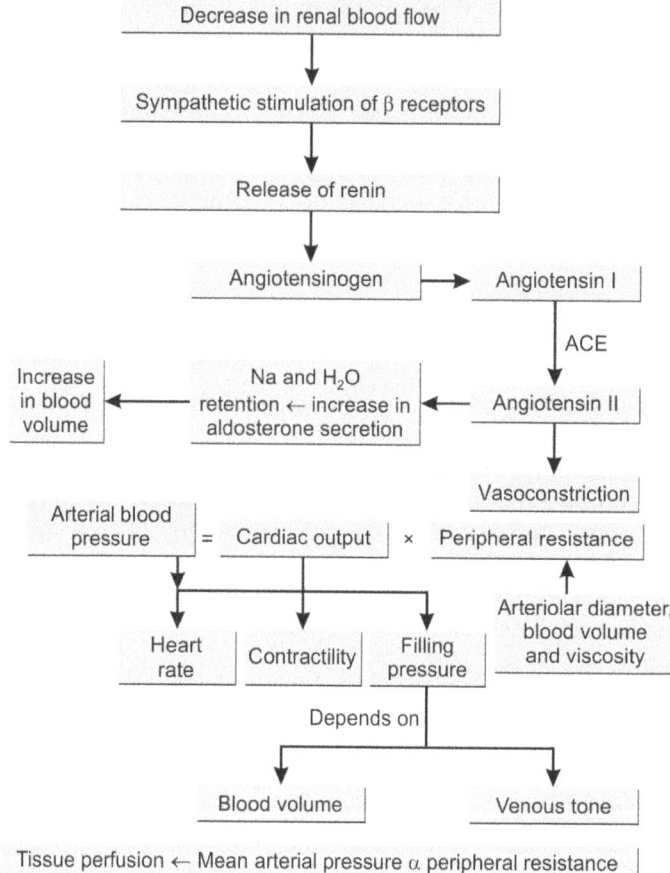

Baroreflexes involve the pressure-sensitive neurons (baroreceptors) in the aortic arch and carotid sinuses and impulses sent to the vasomotor center (VMC) in the medulla. So, fall in BP leads to stimulation of baroreceptors, leading to fewer impulses being sent to vasomotor center, leading to increase in sympathetic and decrease in parasympathetic outflow leading to vasoconstriction and increase in CO.

The kidney provides the long-term control of BP by altering the blood volume (Flowchart 15.4).

TREATMENT

Nondrug regimen: Stop smoking, alcohol, weight reduction, salt restriction, increase in eating fruits or dietary K^+, reduce stress and regular exercise.

Drugs used in Hypertension

- *β-blockers*: Acebutolol, atenolol, betaxolol, bisoprolol, carteolol, carvedilol, esmolol, labetalol, metaprolol, nadolol, pindolol and proprapolol.
- *Centrally acting drugs*: Clonidine, methyldopa and guanabenz.

- Postganglionic sympathetic nerve terminal blockers guanethidine, reserpine and guanadrel.
- $α_1$ *selective blockers*: Doxazosin, prazosin and terazosin.
- *Vasodilators*: Minoxidil, nitroprusside, diazoxide, fenoldopam and hydralazine.
- *Ca-channel blockers*: Amlodipine, felodipine, isradipine, nicardipine, nisoldipine, nifedipine, verapamil and diltiazem.
- *ACE inhibitors*: Benazepril, captopril, enalapril, fosinopril, lisinopril and perindopril.
- *Angiotensin receptors blockers*: Candesartan, losartan, irbesartan, valsartan, telmisartan and olmisartan.
- *New generation centrally acting drug*: Moxonidine.
- *Direct renin inhibitor*: Aliskiren.
- *Diuretics*: Thiazides like chlorthalidone, indapamide, hydrochlorothiazide; Loop diuretics like furosemide, torsemide; potassium-sparing diuretics like amiloride, triamterine.

INDICATIONS FOR THERAPY (TABLE 15.5)

Table 15.5: Classification of hypertension.

Classification	Systolic blood pressure	Diastolic blood pressure
Normal	<120 mm Hg	<80 mm Hg
Prehypertension	120–139 mm Hg	or 80–89 mm Hg
Hypertension stage 1	140–159 mm Hg	or 90–99 mm Hg
Hypertension stage 2	≥160 mm Hg	or ≥100 mm Hg

- Systolic BP >140 mm Hg or diastolic BP >90 mm Hg on several occasions.
- Isolated systolic BP >160 mm Hg specially if aged more than 65 years.
- Diabetic patients or patients with renal disease with BP >130/80 mm Hg.
- Labile hypertension or occasional systolic hypertension to be monitored at 6 monthly interval.

BLOOD PRESSURE MANAGEMENT PROTOCOL

- Preferred initial therapy in stage 1 hypertension is thiazide diuretics. Other drugs recommended are β-blockers, ACE inhibitors/ARBs, Ca-channel antagonists.
- Uncomplicated stage 2 hypertensive patients need an additional drug to diuretics or another class of antihypertensive.
- Presence of complications like heart failure, myocardial infarction, renal failure or associated diabetes pose a challenge to therapy.
- Hypertensive with congestive heart failure (CCF) should be treated with diuretic, β-blocker, angiotensin converting enzyme (ACE) inhibitors ARBs and spironolactone even in absence of hypertension.
- ACE inhibitors or angiotensin receptor blockers (ARBs) should be the first-line antihypertensive therapy in diabetics.

Comparison of commonly used antihypertensive drugs is given in Table 15.6.

Table 15.6: Comparison of commonly used antihypertensives.

Drug	Dose	Indications	Contraindications	Adverse effects	Special comments
1. Diuretics a. Thiazides	Hydrochlorothiazide 125 mg/day, 25 mg orally	CCF, elderly systolic hypertension	Gout, dyslipidemia, sexually active males	Serum electrolyte imbalance hyperglycemia, hyperuricemia, hyperlipidemia	First-line therapy in mild-to-moderate hypertension
b. Loop diuretics	Furosemide 40–240 mg/day, oral, parenteral	Severe hypertension, CCF, cirrhosis	Hyperuriceamia, primary aldosteronism	Hypokalemia, hypomagnesemia, hypocalcemia, rash, dehydration, hypochloremic alkalosis	Recommended in severe hypertension with renal insufficiency when GFR <30–40 mL/min
c. Aldosterone antagonist, spironolactone	50–100 mg/day orally	Hypertension with heart failure, Aldosteronian	Renal failure	Hyperkalemia, gynecomastia	Used in Hypertension due to hypermineralo-corticoidism
d. Potassium-sparing diuretics, Triamterine, amiloride	25–100 mg/day orally, 5–10 mg/day orally, respectively	Hypertension with heart failure, hyperaldosteronism and refractory hypertension	Renal failure	Hyperkalemia, GI symptoms leg cramps, nephrolithiasis	

Contd...

Contd...

Drug	Dose	Indications	Contraindications	Adverse effects	Special comments
Antiadrenergic drugs— a. Centrally acting 1. Clonidine	0.05–0.6 mg oral BD	Mild-to-moderate hypertension with renal disease		Drowsiness/insomnia, postural hypotension, dryness of mouth	Rebound hypertension can occur with abrupt withdrawal, stimulates inhibitory α_2 adrenergic receptors, inhibiting sympathetic outflow
2. Alpha methyl dopa	250–1000 mg BD orally, 250–1000 mg IV 4–6 hourly	Mild-to-moderate hypertension, hypertension in pregnancy	Pheochromocytoma, active hepatic disease	Sedation, postural hypotension, chronic hepatitis, lupus like syndrome	Reduces sympathetic outflow centrally; methyl dopa also used in withdrawal from drug abuse
b. Nerve endings— Guanethidine	10–150 mg orally	Moderate-to-severe hypertension	Pheochromocytoma, severe coronary artery disease, cerebrovascular insufficiency	Postural hypotension, dryness of mouth, bradycardia, fluid retention	Interferes with no-radrenaline release and replaces NA in vessicles
c. Autonomic ganglia – Trimethaphan	1–6 mg/min	Severe-to-malignant hypertension	Severe coronary artery disease, cerebrovascular insufficiency, glaucoma, diabetes	Postural hypotension, dry mouth, constipation, urinary retention, impotence	

Contd...

Contd...

Drug	Dose	Indications	Contraindicactions	Adverse effects	Special comments
d. α$_1$-blockers—Prazosin, terazosin, doxazosin	1–10 mg BD/day, 1–20 mg/day, 1–16 mg/day	Pheochromocytoma, mild-to-moderate hypertension	Severe coronary artery disease, to be used with caution in elderly	Postural hypotension, tachycardia, syncope, fluid retention, miosis, dry mouth	Selectively block α$_1$-receptors leading to vasodilation
e. β-blockers—Propanolol, metaprolol, atenolol, nadolol, bisoprolol	10–120 mg orally twice to 4 times daily, 25–100 mg BD orally, 25–100 mg orally, 20–120 mg orally, 2.5–10 mg orally	Mild-to-moderate hypertension, hyperdynamic circulation	Hyperlipidemia, diabetes, asthma 2nd/3rd degree heart block	Bronchospasm, GI symptoms, fatigue, hyperglycemia, hypercholesterolemia	Labetalol, carvedilol and nebivolol cause less metabolic alteration compared to others
f. Both α$_1$ and β-receptor blockers, labetolol, carvedilol	100–400 mg BD orally, 10–80 mg IV every 10 min, 12.5–50 mg orally daily in divided doses	Do Hypertensive emergency Do	As above	As above more incidence of postural hypotension, less incidence of metabolic alterations	

Contd...

Contd...

Drug	Dose	Indications	Contraindicactions	Adverse effects	Special comments
Vasodilators 1. Hydralazine 2. Minoxidil 3. Diazoxide 4. Nitroprusside	1. Oral 10-75 mg 4 times IV/IM 10–50 mg 6 hourly 25–40 mg BD 2. Orally 1–3 mg/kg IV 3. Max 150 mg, 0.5–8 µg/kg/min IV	1. Moderate-to-severe hypertension 2. Severe hypertension 3. Severe-or-malignant hypertension, 4. Malignant hypertension	SLE, severe coronary A disease Diabetic, hyperuricaemia, CCF	1. Lupus like syndrome, tachycardia 2. Tachycardia, hair growth on face and body, coarsening of facial features, fluid retention, pericardial effusion 3. Hyperglycemia, hyperuricemia, sodium retention 4. Nausea and vomiting, weakness, apprehension, cyanide toxicity	1. Decrease diastolic BP > systolic BP, arterioles > veins 2. Hypertrichosis creates a problem
ACE Inhibitors 1. Captopril 2. Ramipril 3. Enalapril 4. Enalaprilat 5. Lisinopril ARBs 1 Losartan, 2 Valsartan	1. 12.5–75 mg BD orally 2. 1.25–20 mg daily orally 3. 2.5–40 mg orally 0.625–1.25 mg 4. IV over 5 min, 6–8 hourly 5–40 mg orally, 5. 25–50 mg BD orally, 80–320 mg orally	Mild to severe hypertension, hypertension with diabetes or heart failure, diabetic nephropathy, history of MI, non-diabetic proteinuria	Pregnancy, bilateral, renal, artery stenosis, renal failure, severe aortic stenosis	Cough, angioedema, urticaria, dysgeusia, hyperkalemia, leukopeia, pancytopemia, teratogenicity, ARBs have similar profile except that incidence of cough (due to bradykinin) is minimum	Inhibit ACE, decrease in Angiotensin II level, decrease in vasoconstriction, In acute severe hypertension, sublingual (chewed) captopril can rapidly bring down BP

Contd...

Contd...

Drug	Dose	Indications	Contraindicactions	Adverse effects	Special comments
Calcium channel blockers 1. Nifedipine 2. Amlodipine 3. Nicardipine, 4. Diltiazem 5. Verapanil	1. 30–90 mg daily orally 2. 2.5–10 mg daily orally 3. 20–40 mg 3 times daily orally 4. 30–90 mg 4 times daily 5. 30–120 mg 4 times daily	Hypertensive patients with angina, elderly patients systolic hypertension, peripheral vascular disease, mild to moderate hypertension	Heart failure, heart block	Tachycardia, flushing, GI effects pedal edema, constipation, headache	Dihydropyridines like amlodipine are commonly preferred, tachycardia/edema does not occur with diltiazen but liver dysfunction can occur. Phenylalkylamine, verapanil is commonly used in arrhythmias

Management of anesthesia for hypertensive patients include:
- Assessment of extent of disease.
- Evaluation of drug therapy.
- Preparation for exaggerated BP rise during operation and prophylactic use of β-blockers or clonidine in hypertensive patients, IHD patients, in peripheral vascular disease, coronary artery disease or hypercholesterolemia may decrease perioperative death rate.

Moxonidine
- New generation centrally acting antihypertensive.
- Selective agonist at the imidazoline receptor subtype 1 (1_1).
- Causes decrease in sympathetic activity and decreases BP.
- Indicated in treatment of mild to moderate essential hypertension.

Table 15.7: Antihypertensives in special conditions.

Concomitant disease	First choice	Second choice
1. Angina pectoris	β Blockers, Ca channel antagonists	Diuretics
2. Diabetes	ACE inhibitors, Ca channel antagonists	Ca-channel blockers
3. Hyperlipidemia	ACE inhibitors, Ca channel antagonists	
4. CHF	Diuretics, ACE inhibitors	Avoid Ca-channel blockers
5. Previous MI	β blockers, ACE inhibitors	Diuretics, Ca-channel blockers
6. Chronic renal disease	Diuretics	β blockers, ACE inhibitors
7. Asthma or COPD	Diuretics	ACE inhibitors

Points to note—(evidence based)
- Alpha 2 agonists may reduce the incidence of perioperative cardiac events of major surgery.
- Pretreatment with β-blocker, e.g. esmolol or α_2-agonist, clonidine blunts excessive sympathetic response during surgery.
- The duration of direct laryngoscopy should be <15 seconds; in addition laryngotracheal lignocaine immediately before placement of endotracheal tube, minimizes pressor response.
- Regional anesthesia is preferred in patients with congestive heart failure where β-blockers are rather contraindicated.
- Antihypertensives are also used in some special conditions such as, angina pectoris, diabetes, etc. (Table 15.7).

DRUGS USED IN ISCHEMIC HEART DISEASE

INTRODUCTION

- Stable angina → Treatment goal, increase in myocardial O_2 demand (increase in O_2 demand with exertion).
- Unstable angina → Treatment goal, increase in myocardial blood flow, antiplatelet agents, heparin, coronary, stents/bypass surgery (increase in O_2 demand due to decrease in blood supply, e.g. thrombosis).
- Vasospasm of coronary vessels → Treatment goal, increase in myocardial blood flow, antiplatelet agents, heparin (Prinzmetal angina). Drugs used in angina may provide prophylactic or symptomatic treatment but β receptor antagonists also reduce mortality except in Prinzmetal angina. ACE inhibitors also decrease mortality.

DRUGS USED IN ANGINA

- *Nitrates*: Nitroglycerine, Isosorbide dinitrate, Isosorbide mononitrate.
- β-blockers.
- Ca-channel blockers.
- K^+ channel openers, e.g. nicorandil.
- *Others*: Antiplatelet drugs (aspirin, clopidogrel), lipid-lowering agents (statins), intracoronary drug eluting stents (paciltaxel, sirolimus).
    - Major determinants of myocardial O_2 consumption—Left ventricular wall tension, heart rate and myocardial contractility.
    - Ventricular wall tension → is dependent on preload (ventricular end-diastolic pressure) and afterload (peripheral resistance).

DRUG THERAPY IN ACUTE MYOCARDIAL INFARCTION

Immediate Therapy

- *Supportive*:
    - To alley pain, anxiety and apprehension—opioid analgesics—morphine/pethidine and diazepam.
    - Humidified O_2.
    - Maintenance of blood volume, tissue perfusion and microcirculation—IV infusion, and Correction of acidosis—sodium bicarbonate IV.
    - Sublingual nitroglycerine; low dose aspirin (160–325 mg) to be chewed or swallowed immediately.
    - β-blocker, e.g. metoprolol infusion for few days → decrease in infarct size and complications.
- *Treatment of pump failure*:
    - Furosemide/loop diuretic
    - Glyceryl trinitrate/nitroprusside/ACE inhibitor/vasodilator.
    - Ionotropic agent—Dopamine/Dobutamine.
    - Heparin followed by oral anticoagulant.
    - Thrombolysis by streptokinase/urokinase/alteplase.

- ACE inhibitors—to prevent remodeling of heart or precipitation of heart failure.

Prevention of Future Attack
- Platelet function inhibitors—aspirin, clopidogrel.
- β-blockers—if not contraindicated, continued for two years.
- Control of hyperlipidemia—statins.
- Pathophysiology of myocardial ischaemia in shown in Figure 15.3.

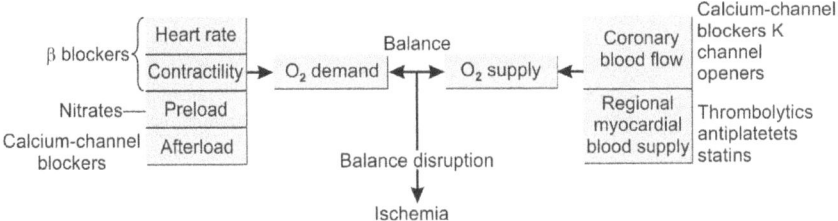

Figure 15.3: Pathophysiology of myocardial ischemia and its treatment.

CLINICAL PEARL

- Inhaled NO exerts its therapeutic effects on pulmonary vasculature and is used to treat pulmonary hypertension, specially in hypoxemic neonates. It reduces both morbidity and mortality.
- Nitrous oxide may increase pulmonary vascular resistance and is avoided.
- *Drugs used in pulmonary hypertension*:
  - Prostaglandins—epoprostenol, iloprost, treprostinil
  - Endothelin receptor antagonists—bosentan, sitaxsentan, ambrisentan
  - Inhaled nitric oxide, inhaled milrinone
  - Type V phosphodiesterase inhibitors—sildenafil, vardenafil
  - Soluble guanylate cyclase activators—cinaciguat, riociguat.

DIURETICS

Diuretics increase urine output with increased sodium excretion. They are the first-line drug therapy for hypertension and used for symptomatic relief in heart failure with fluid retention (Tables 15.8 to 15.10).

Table 15.8: Mechanism of action and uses of commonly used diuretics.

Diuretics	Mechanism of action (Fig. 15.4)	Main uses
1. Thiazides (moderate-efficacy diuretics)	Site of action is the cortical diluting segment at initial part of distal tubule. Acts by inhibiting Na^+, Cl^- symport, receptors being located at the luminal membrane	Mild to moderate hypertension, mild to moderate edema, hypercalciuria, diabetes insipidus (DI)
2. Loop diuretics (high ceiling diuretics)	Site of action is the thick ascending segment of loop of Henle. Acts by inhibiting Na^+, K^+, Cl^- cotransport. Has weak inhibitory action on renal carbonic anhydrase	Cardiac, hepatic or renal edema, acute left ventricular failure (LVF), pulmonary edema, cerebral edema, hypertensive crisis
3. Potassium-sparing diuretics	Site of action is latter part of distal tubule and CD where renal epithelial sodium channels are present. These Na^+ channels are blocked from the luminal side, decrease luminal negative transmembrane potential, which controls K^+ and H^+ secretion	Usually used along with thiazide or loop diuretics
4. Aldosterone antagonists (weak diuretics)	Site of action latter part of distal tubule and collecting duct (CD) cells. Acts by binding to mineralocorticoid receptor (MR) prevents action of aldosterone, preventing synthesis of aldosterone-induced proteins thereby preventing activation of Na^+ channels	Edema of nephrotic syndrome and cirrhosis. Along with thiazide or loop diuretics, CHF

Table 15.9: Comparison of diuretics.

Drug	Dose/day	Indications	Contra-indicactions	Adverse effects	Special comments
1. Diuretics a. Thiazides	Hydrochlorothiazide 12.5–25 mg orally	CCF, elderly systolic hypertension	Gout, dyslipidemia, sexually active males	Serum electrolyte imbalance hyperglycemia, hyperuricemia, hyperlipidemia	First-line therapy in mild to moderate hypertension
b. Loop diuretics	Furosemide 40–240 mg/day, oral, parenteral	Severe hypertension, CCF, cirrhosis	Hyperuricemia, primary aldosteronism	Hypokalemia, hypomagnesemia, hypocalcemia rash, dehydration, hypochloremic alkalosis	Recommended in severe hyper-tension with renal insufficiency when GFR < 30–40 mL/min

Contd...

Contd...

Drug	Dose/day	Indications	Contra-indicactions	Adverse effects	Special comments
c. Aldosterone antagonist, spironolactone	50–100 mg/day orally	Hypertension with heart failure, aldosteronian	Renal failure	Hyperkalemia, gynecomastia	Used in hypertension due to hypermineralocorticoidism
d. Potassium sparing diuretics, triamterene, amiloride	25–100 mg/day orally, 5–10 mg/day orally	Hypertension with heart failure, aldosteronian	Renal failure	Hyperkalemia, GI symptoms leg cramps, nephrolithiasis	

Table 15.10: Doses of commonly used diuretics.

	Dose/day	Remarks
1. Thiazides		
a. Hydrochlorothiazide	12.5–25 mg oral	12.5 mg good for control of hypertension
b. Chlorthalidone	12.5–25 mg oral	12.5 mg good for control of hypertension
c. Bendrofluazide		Higher doses like 25 mg increase the risk of development of diabetes
d. Indapamide	1.5 sustained release (SR) tablet/day mg or 2.5 mg orally	Thiazides except metolazone are not effective at glomerular filtration rate (GFR) < 20–30
e. Metolazone	5–20 mg daily	8–10 hours duration
2. Loop diuretics		Active in patients even with renal failure
a. Furosemide	20–80 mg oral	Quick onset of action (5–10 min if parenteral, 20–30 min if given orally)
b. Bumetanide	0.5–2 mg oral	All loop diuretics except ethacrynic A are sulfonamides
c. Torsemide	5–20 mg oral	
d. Ethacrynic acid	50–200 mg oral	Hence allergic skin, rash, eosinophilia can occur. Long-term use → distal nephron hypertrophy; resistance seen in advanced chronic renal failure (CRF), congestive heart failure CHF, nephrotic syndrome
3. Potassium-sparing D		
a. Amiloride	5 mg	Not metabolized, longer duration of action
b. Triamterene	50–100 mg	Extensively metabolized, shorter duration of action
c. Spironolactone	25–100 mg tab	Slow onset of action
d. Eplerenone	Used only for hypertension	More selective action on mineralocorticoid receptor (MI), less side effects

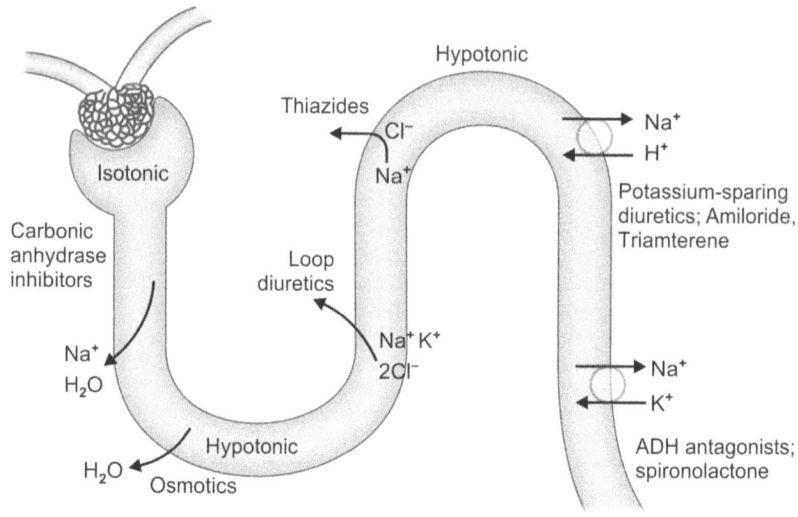

Figure 15.4: Sites of action of diuretics.

OSMOTIC DIURETICS

Relatively inert pharmacological agents, which are freely filtered through the glomerulus and undergo limited reabsorption in the renal tubule. Being osmotically active, they inhibit osmosis of water into the interstitial space and also reduce Na⁺ reabsorption. Major site of action is the proximal tubule and descending loop of Henle. Mannitol is the prototype drug. Others—glycerol, isosorbide and urea.

Glycerol and isosorbide can be given orally. Urea and mannitol are given intravenously.

Mechanism of Action

Acts primarily by increasing extracellular osmolality, thereby extracting water from the intracellular space. As they are not metabolized, they are freely filtered through the glomerulus and prevent absorption of water due to its osmotic action. Thereby urine volume increases. Sodium reabsorption is also affected as the contact time of tubular fluid is lessened. As the natriuresis is less compared to the diuresis, there may be resultant hypovolemia but relative hypernatremia. Increased GFR reduces renin release. Along with Na⁺ loss, there is also urinary excretion of other anions and cations like K⁺, Cl⁻, and HCO_3^-.

Uses

- Increased intracranial tension or cerebral edema.
- Increased intraocular tension.

- Acute renal failure to maintain GFR.
- Dialysis disequilibrium syndrome [too rapid removal of solutes from extracellular fluid (ECF) due to hemodialysis leads to decrease in osmolality of ECF].
- Neurosurgery to prevent or treat cerebral edema.

Dose

Test dose of 12.5 IV followed by 12.5-25 g IV to maintain GFR of 100 mL. per hour. For increased ICT, 1-2 g/kg of mannitol is administered IV. Therapeutic action must take place within 60-90 minutes. Mannitol should not be used chronically.
- *Contraindications*: Acute tubular necrosis, anuria, chronic heart failure, pulmonary edema, cerebral hemorrhage.
- *Side effect*: Headache, nausea and vomiting, electrolyte imbalances, especially hypo/hypernatremia.

Monitoring of patient during mannitol therapy is essential as overuse of mannitol without adequate fluid replacement may result in dehydration, hyperkalemia and hypernatremia.

VASOPRESSIN ANTAGONISTS

Active in conditions where water retention occurs due to antidiuretic hormone (ADH) excess.
- Vaptans, e.g. conivaptan, tolvaptan and mozavaptan.
- Tetracycline group of drug demeclocycline.

Mechanism of Action

Conivaptan acts as antagonist at V_1a and V_2 receptors. Lithium and demeclocycline inhibit formation of c AMP in response to ADH. V_2 receptor antagonists or aquaretics increase renal excretion of water without affecting electrolyte excretion.

Uses

SIADH, nephrogenic, diabetes insipidus and CHF.

Toxicity

Renal failure, chronic interstitial nephritis, hepatotoxicity and drug interactions.

PATHOPHYSIOLOGY OF RENIN–ANGIOTENSIN SYSTEM

The renin-angiotensin system participates significantly in the pathophysiology of—hypertension, congestive heart failure, myocardial infarction and diabetic nephropathy.

Hence, the study of the renin–angiotensin system becomes a necessity.

COMPONENTS OF RENIN-ANGIOTENSIN SYSTEM

A. *Renin*: Acid protease secreted by the kidneys into the bloodstream. The secretion of renin from the JG cells is controlled by:
   i. Macula densa cells: Increase NaCl flux—inhibit release, decrease in NaCl flux—stimulate renin,
   ii. Adenosine via A_1 adenosine receptor inhibits renin release.
   iii. PGs stimulate renin release (COX 2 inhibition → blocks macula densa-mediated renin release).
   iv. nNOS inhibition decrease in renin release. There is a biochemical interplay between COX 2, and n NOS in the regulation of macula-densa mediated renin release.
   v. Intrarenal baroreceptor pathway—increase in preglomerular blood vessels → decrease in renin. Decrease in preglomerular blood vessels → increase in renin release,
   vi. β receptor pathway mediated by the release of NE from post-ganglionic sympathetic nerve endings. Activation of $β_1$ receptors → on JG cells release of renin.

   Inhibition of renin release is mediated by: (a) stimulation of AT_1 receptors by angiotensin II (short loop negative feedback), (b) activation of baroreceptors due to increase in sympathetic tone (long loop negative feedback).

   Physiological and pharmacological parameters influencing renin release:
   - Arterial blood pressure.
   - Dietary salt intake.
   - Loop diuretics.
   - NSAIDs.
   - ACE inhibitors.
   - ARBs.
   - β-blockers.
   - Phosphodiesterase inhibitors.
   - Vasodilators.

B. *Angiotensinogen*:
   - An abundant globular glycoprotein.
   - MW-55,000–60,000.
   - Substrate of renin.
   - Synthesized primarily in liver; also found in fat, certain regions in CNS and kidney.

- Circulating level of angiotensinogen is increased by—inflammation, insulin, estrogen, glucocorticoid, thyroid hormone, several cytokines and angiotensin II.

  A missense mutation in the angiotensinogen gene that increases plasma level of angiotensinogen is associated with essential hypertension and pregnancy-induced hypertension.

C. *Angiotensin-converting enzyme (Flowchart 15.5):*
   - An ectoenzyme and glycoprotein.
   - MW-170000.
   - Human ACE has 2 homologous domains, each with a catalytic site and a Zn-binding region.
   - ACE is nonspecific and cleaves dipeptide units from substrates with diverse amino acid sequences.
   - ACE is identical to kininase II, enzyme that inactivates bradykinin and other potent vasodilator peptides.

   Angiotensin-converting enzyme are of 2 types: (1) Somatic—found throughout the body; (2) Germinal: found in postmeiotic spermatogenic cells and spermatozoa.

   Many tissues including the brain, pituitary, blood vessels, heart, kidney, adrenal gland exhibit local renin-angiotensin systems, independent of renal/hepatic-based system.

   Local production of angiotensin II by intrinsic local renin angiotensin system may influence vascular, cardiac and renal function and structure.

   Non-ACE angiotensin I processing enzymes, e.g. cathepsin G, chymase etc. contribute to the local tissue conversion of angiotensin I to angiotensin II especially in the heart.

D. *Angiotensin peptides are of three types:* Angiotensin I, angiotensin II, angiotensin III.

   Angiotensin I is less than 1% potent as angiotensin II on smooth muscles, heart and adrenal cortex. Angiotensin II and angiotensin III cause quantitative similar effects and stimulate aldosterone with equal potency but angiotensin III is 25% as potent as angiotensin II in elevating BP, and 10% as potent in stimulating the adrenal medulla. Angiotensin II is rapidly destroyed (1-2 min) resulting heptapeptide is angiotensin III.

   Functions:
   - Potent vasoconstrictor: Increase in both systolic and diastolic BP.
   - Increase in secretion of aldosterone by acting or adrenal cortex.
   - Act on the brain to increase in BP and water intake.

E. *Angiotensin receptors:* There are 2 subtypes → AT_1
   $\searrow AT_2$

   These are heptahelical G-protein coupled receptors (GPCRs).

   Most of the known biological effects of angiotensin II are mediated by AT_1 receptors. Functional role of AT_2 receptors is poorly defined but though it is conceptualized as cardiovascular protective receptor, it may contribute to cardiac fibrosis.

Functions and Effects of the Renin-Angiotensin System

1. Angiotensin II is a potent vasoconstrictor → altered peripheral resistance—constricts precapillary arterioles and postcapillary venules to a lesser extent, vasoconstrictor strongest in the kidneys → splanchnic bed → brain → lungs → skeletal muscles. Decreases cerebral and coronary blood flow, enhances peripheral noradrenergic neurotransmission by:
   - Inhibiting reuptake of NE
   - Augmenting NE release
   - Enhancing vascular response of NE
   - CNS is affected by both locally formed and blood-borne angiotensin II.
   - Increase in sympathetic tone.
   - Release of ADH from neurohypophysis.
   - Dipsogenic effect: Release of catecholamine from adrenal medulla.
2. Altered renal function:
   - Decrease in urinary excretion of Na^+ and H_2O
   - Increase in K^+ excretion

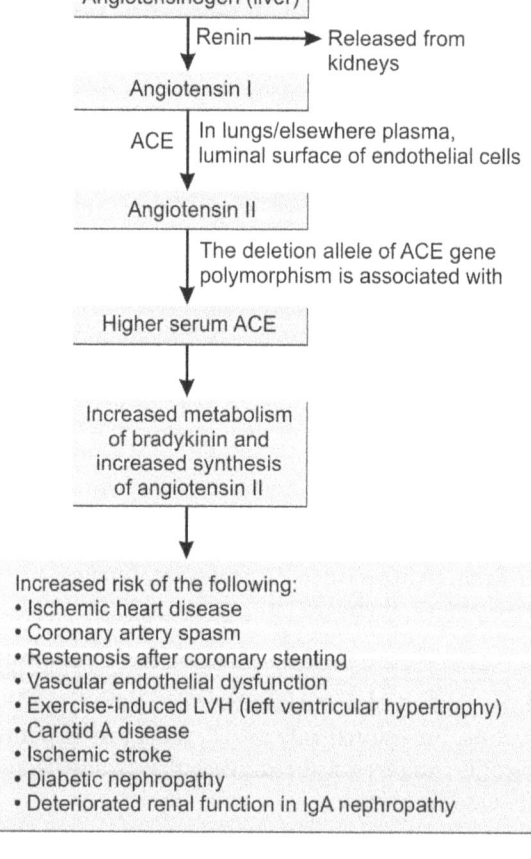

Flowchart 15.5: Mechanism of action of renin-angiotensin system.

- Shifts renal pressure – natriuresis curve to right
- Stimulates Na^+/H^+ exchange in the proximal tubule. So increase in reabsorption of Na^+, Cl^+ and HCO_3^-.
- Stimulates $Na^+/K^+/2\,Cl$ symporter in the thick ascending limb of nephron.
- Stimulates zona glomerulosa of adrenal cortex to release aldosterone.
- Altered renal hemodynamics influences GFR.

3. Alteration of cardiovascular structure:
   - Concentric cardiac hypertrophy
   - Eccentric cardiac hypertrophy
   - Increase in wall lumen ratio of blood vessels
   - Thickening of intimal surface of blood vessels.

   Angiotensin II stimulates migration, proliferation, hypertrophy and/or synthetic capacity of vascular smooth muscle cells, cardiac myocytes and fibroblasts.

4. Other effects: Marked anorexigenic effect and weight loss.

ACE INHIBITORS

- Teprotide → 1st ACE inhibitor obtained from pit viper venom; not used due to brief duration of action and parenteral administration.
- Other drugs which are orally active:
  - *Captopril*: duration of action 6–12 hours but quick onset of action.
  - *Enalapril*: Enalaprilat can be used IV.
  - *Lisinopril*: Active drug and lysine derivative of enalaprilat.
  - *Ramipril*: Inhibit renin-angiotensin system (RAS) to greater extent and extensive tissue distribution.
  - *Fosinopril*: Eliminated both by liver and kidney.
  - *Perindopril*: Long-acting but onset of action slow.

CHARACTERISTICS

- All are prodrugs except captopril and lisinopril.
- Bioavailability maximum with captopril—minimum with perindopril.
- Greater fall in BP in renovascular, accelerated and malignant hypertension; effects variable in essential hypertension.
- Decrease in peripheral resistance is mainly responsible for fall in BP.
- Both systolic and diastolic BP decrease but no effect on CO and cardiovascular reflexes.
- Mainly arterioles dilate, increase in compliance of larger arteries but little effect on capacitance vessels.
- Reflex sympathetic stimulation does not occur in spite of vasodilation.
- Renal blood flow is not compromised even in case of hypotension.
- Increase in level of plasma renin and angiotensin-I (A-I) but not of physiological significance.
- Basal levels of aldosterone is decreased.
- Food alters bioavailability, excreted via urine.
- Duration of action more than 14 hours except captopril.

ADVERSE EFFECTS (FIG. 15.5)

(a) Hypotension, (b) brassy cough, (c) urticaria and rash, (d) angioedema, (e) dysgeusia, (f) fetopathic effect, and (g) hyperkalemia.

Co-administration of following drugs should be avoided:
  i. K^+-sparing diuretics
  ii. Nonsteroidal anti-inflammatory drugs (NSAIDs)
  iii. Antacid
  iv. Lithium.

Uses

Hypertension, CHF, MI, diabetic nephropathy and scleroderma crisis.

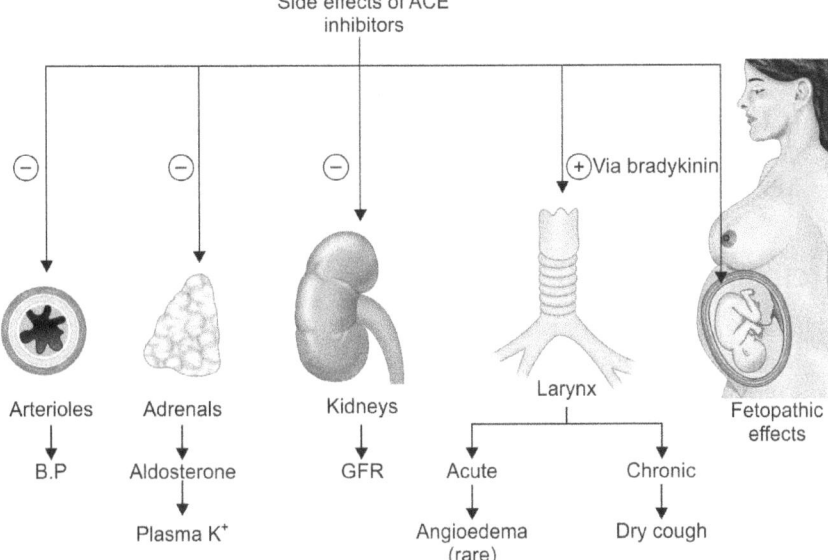

Figure 15.5: Schematic diagram showing side effects of ACE inhibitors.

ANGIOTENSIN II RECEPTOR BLOCKERS (ARBs)

- Losartan and other AT receptor antagonists:
  - *Candesartan*: Eliminated by both liver and kidney.
  - *Valsartan*: Food interferes with absorption.
  - *Telmisartan*: Excreted unchanged in bile.
  - *Irbesartan*: High oral BA and excreted via bile.

ACTIONS

- More selective blocker of AT_1 than AT_2.
- Block all actions of A-II, e.g. vasoconstrictor central and peripheral sympathetic stimulations, release of aldosterone, release of adrenaline from adrenals, release of ADH, prevent growth-promoting actions on heart and blood vessels.

ADVANTAGES

- Does not interfere with degradation of bradykinin—cough does not occur.
- Even if A-II is produced by alternative pathways, especially in tissues → ARBs block its actions.
- Lower incidence of side effects, e.g. cough, rash, angioedema, dysgeusia.

CHARACTERISTICS

- Orally active but poor BA.
- Highly protein bound in plasma.
- Excreted mostly via bile.
  - *Side effect*: Minimum—headache, dizziness, weakness mild gastrointestinal (GI) effects.
  - *Indications*: As ACE inhibitors.
  - *Contraindication*: Pregnancy.

CALCIUM CHANNEL BLOCKERS

Three subclasses of calcium channel antagonists are present (Table 15.11):
- Phenylalkylamine derivatives—Verapamil.
- Dihydropyridines (DHPs)—Amlodipine, felodipine, isradipine, nicardipine, nifedipine, nisoldipine, cilnidipine.
- Benzothiazepines—Diltiazem.

MECHANISM OF ACTION (TABLES 15.12 TO 15.14)

These agents modify the entry of calcium into specific cells by binding to α, subunit of L-type of voltage-dependent calcium channels. Each class has

Table 15.11: Types of calcium channels.

Ca channel	Sites	Blocked by
L	Cardiac muscles, smooth muscles, endocrine cells, neurons, bone	Verapamil, DHPs
T	Heart, neurons	Flunarizine
N	Neurons, sperm	Ziconotide, gabapentin
P/Q	Neurons	
R	Neurons, sperm	

Table 15.12: Actions of calcium channel blockers.

Sites of blockade		Action	Remarks
1. Smooth muscles	Blood vessels	Most sensitive, relaxation, arterioles > veins	Decrease in coronary A tone, decrease in peripheral resistance
	Bronchiolar	Relaxation	
	Gastrointestinal	Relaxation	May result in constipation
	Uterine	Relaxation	
2. Cardiac muscles		Decrease in contraction	Negative inotropic action (DHPs)
SA node and AV node		Decrease in conduction	Decrease in tachycardia (verapamil, diltiazem)
3. Cerebral blood vessels following subarachnoid hemorrhage		Decrease in cerebral vasospasm	Decrease in cerebral damage following cardiovascular accident (CVA) (nicardipine, nimodipine)
4. P- glycoprotein of cancer cells		Reverse drug resistance	Useful in cancer chemotherapy (verapamil)

Note: DHPs act preferentially on vessels > myocardium > node. Non-DHPs act preferentially on SA and AV nodes > myocardium = vessels.

Table 15.13: Comparison of actions of commonly used calcium channel blockers.

Parameter	Verapamil	Nifedipine	Diltiazem
Heart rate	↓	↑	↓
AV conduction rate	↓↓	—	↓
Contractility	—↓	↓	↓↑
Cardiac output	↓	↓↑	↑

Table 15.14: Calcium channel blockers compared.

Drug	Dose	Indications
A. Dihydropyridines		
1. Amlodipine	Dose of amlodipine 5–10 mg orally OD 20–40 mg 3 times daily orally;	Angina, hypertension
2. Nifedipine	3–10 µg/kg IV	Angina, hypertension, Raynaud's phenomenon
3. Felodipine	5–10 mg orally OD	Hypertension, Raynaud's phenomenon
4. Nicardipine	20–40 mg orally 8 hourly	Angina, hypertension
5. Nimodipine	40 mg orally 4 hourly	Subarachnoid hemorrhage
B. Non-dihydropyridines		
1. Diltiazem	30–80 mg orally 6 hourly, 75–150 µg/kg IV	Angina, hypertension, Raynaud's phenomenon
2. Verapamil	80–160 mg orally 8 hourly, 75–150 µg/kg IV	Angina, hypertension, arrhythmia, migraine

specific binding sites which are variably expressed in various tissues. All calcium channel blockers are vasodilators but reflex tachycardia is caused by the dihydropyridines. Verapamil and diltiazem depress the SA node and AV conduction system of the heart and have negative inotropic action. Neurons with L-type channels, however, are less sensitive.

Other types of calcium channels are less sensitive to blockade so cardiac and smooth muscles are affected rather than neurons and secretory glands.

- *Pharmacokinetics*: Orally administered 90–100% absorption. BA variable due to high first pass metabolism except amlodipine. High plasma protein binding (minimum diltiazem, maximum felodipine), > 90% metabolized in liver.
- *Uses*: Hypertension, angina, hypertropic cardiomyopathy and cardiac arrhythmias.
- *Side effect*: Palpitation, flushing, ankle edema, headache and drowsiness.

- *Contraindications*: Post-MI patients, elderly males with prostatic hypertrophy and uncontrolled diabetes.

VERAPAMIL

Phenylalkylamine mainly used for the treatment and prophylaxis of paroxysmal supraventricular tachycardia (PSVT). First to be synthesized as analogue of papaverine, vasodilator alkaloid obtained from poppy seeds.

Uses

1. Treatment and prevention of SVT
2. Treatment of hypertension
3. Prophylaxis of angina

Though it can be used in hypertension and angina, there are better drugs, mainly used in SVT.

- *Actions*: Negative inotropic and chronotropic; main action is on cardiac conduction.
- *Use*: Given in slow bolus injection (5-10 mg) over 2-3 minutes to terminate SVT. A further dose of 5 mg can be given after 5-10 minutes. As prophylaxis, 40-120 mg is given TDS orally.
- *Side effect*: (1) Hypotension, (2) precipitation of heart failure, (3) bradycardia (hence slow IV), (4) gynecomastia, and (5) gingival hyperplaxia.

Precautions during use:
- Cardiac monitoring.
- Prior BP measurement and pulse rate recording.
  - Contraindications
    - LVF or CHF.
    - Second or third degree heart block
    - Sick sinus syndrome
    - β-blocker coadministration
    - Severe liver impairment
  - Advantage: It can be used in asthma patients in whom adenosine is contraindicated.
  - Drug interactions: (1) β-blockers, (2) digoxin, (3) cyclosporin and (4) grapefruit juice.

CILNIDIPINE

Novel Ca-channel antagonist which blocks both L-type and N-type calcium channels. Used as antihypertensive. Advantages: Dilate both arterioles and venules.
- Long half-life, hence once daily dose is sufficient.
- Less incidence of reflex tachycardia, pedal edema.

CARDIAC GLYCOSIDES

Drugs which consist of an aglycone and one or more sugar moieties. These drugs have increased cardiac inotropic action without altering the O_2 consumption. The pharmacological activity resides in the aglycone and consists of a cyclopentanoperhydrophenanthrene ring (Tables 15.15 and 15.16).

Table 15.15: Cardiac glycosides.

Glycoside	Its source
1. Digitoxin	Digitalis purpurea, digitalis lanata
2. Digoxin	Digitalis lanata
3. Strophanthin G	Strophanthus gratus
4. Thevetia	Thevetia nerüfolia

Table 15.16: Differences between digitoxin and digoxin.

	Digoxin	Digitoxin
Onset of action	15–30 min	30–60 min
Duration of action	2–5 hours	6–12 hours
Route of administration	IV, oral	Oral
Oral absorption	60–80%	90–100%
Use	Emergency	Maintenance
Plasma ther. conc.	15–30 mg/mL	0.5–1.4 mg/mL
Route of excretion	Renal	Hepatic

MECHANISM OF ACTION

Both therapeutic and toxic effects of digitalis are due to myocardial Ca^{+2} loading (Flowchart 15.6).

Flowchart 15.6: Mechanism of action of cardiac glycosides.

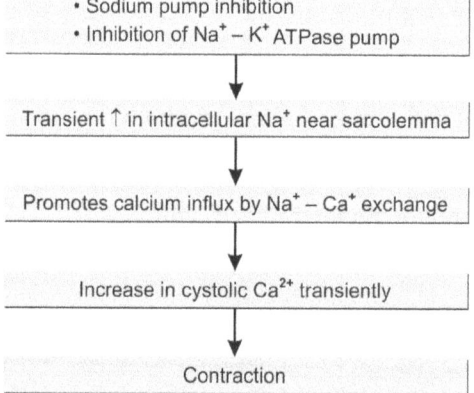

Pharmacokinetics of Digoxin
- About 75% of oral dose is absorbed, rest is inactivated in lower gut.
- Circulated in blood, unbound to plasma protein.
- Binds to tissues, receptors in heart and skeletal muscles.
- Lipid-soluble.
- Excreted unchanged in urine.

Effects
- Weak inotropic effect.
- Slows ventricular rate especially in atrial fibrillation.
- Decreases sympathetic drive.
- Sinus slowing and AV nodal inhibition.
- Action of digoxin on AV conduction prolongs refractory period.
- Renin release from the kidney is inhibited.
- Mild direct vasoconstrictor action as reflex sympathetic overactivity is withdrawn → net decrease in peripheral resistance.
- No prominent effect on BP; pulse may increase.

High serum digoxin level occurs in severe hypokalemia, depressed renal blood flow, depressed GFR, concurrent therapy with quinidine, verapamil, amiodarone, calcium channel blockers, antibiotics, e.g. erythromycin and tetracycline.

Precautions
(1) Hypokalemia, (2) elderly, renal or hepatic disease, (3) MI, (4) thyrotoxicosis, (5) myxedema, (6) ventricular tachycardia, (7) partial AV block, and (8) WPW syndrome.

Disadvantages of Digoxin Therapy
- Narrow therapeutic window, preferable to maintain plasma concentration below 1 mg/mL, especially < 0.8 mg/mL (0.5–1 mg/mL).
- Several drug interactions.
- Altered electrolyte balance may precipitate toxicity.

Contraindications
(1) HOCM, (2) renal dysfunction, (3) WPW syndrome, (4) AV nodal block, and (5) diastolic dysfunction.

Features of Digitalis Toxicity
- Anorexia, nausea, vomiting and diarrhea.
- Malaise, fatigue, confusion, insomnia, yellow or green halos.
- Palpitation and arrhythmia, syncope.
- Blood levels showing increase in digoxin level, low potassium level, magnesium, urea and creatinine.

Uses
- CHF, atrial flutter (AF), atrial fibrillation and PSVT.

CARDIAC DYSRHYTHMIA AND ANTIARRHYTHMICS

- Disturbances of cardiac impulse conduction.
- Classified according to the site of conduction block relative to the AV node.
- Heart block above the AV node—benign and transient.
- Heart block below the AV node—progressive and permanent types.

FIRST-DEGREE AV HEART BLOCK

- *Definition*: PR interval on ECG > 0.2 sec at a heart rate of 70/min.
- *Pathology*: Delay in passage of cardiac impulse through AV node.
- *Cause*: Degenerative change due to aging (commonest cause), digitalis, ischemia of AV node, enhanced parasympathetic activity associated with AI (usually asymptomatic).
- *Treatment*: IV atropine.

SECOND-DEGREE AV HEART BLOCK

- Two types: Mobitz type I block (Wenckebach).
- Cause: Delayed conduction of cardiac impulse through AV node with progressive prolongation of PR interval until a beat is entirely blocked (dropped beat) followed by a repeat of the sequence.
- Mobitz type II block: Reflects disease in His-Purkinje conduction system (infranodal) characterized by sudden interruption of cardiac impulse without prior prolongation of P-R in ECG.
- Type 2 has a more serious prognosis as it often progresses to third degree AV heart block.
- Treatment type 2 block may include placement of an artificial cardiac pacemaker.

Unifascicular Heart Block

Block of conduction of cardiac impulse over the left anterior/posterior fascicle of left bundle branch → unifascicular block or hemiblock.

Block of left anterior fascicle of left bundle branch—left anterior hemiblock. Left posterior hemiblock is uncommon as the posterior fascicle is larger and better perfused. ECG change—QRS complex may be normal or only minimally prolonged.

Right Bundle Branch Block (RBBB)

Block in conduction through right bundle branch is present in 1% of hospitalized patient. ECG change—QRS complex exceeding 0.1 sec and broad RSR complex in V_1, V_3 leads. RBBB does not always imply cardiac disease and is often of no clinical significance.

Left Bundle Branch Block (LBBB)

The LBBB is recognized on ECG as a QRS complex > 0.12 sec in duration and wide notched R waves in all leads. LBBB is often associated with ischemic heart disease, left ventricular hypertrophy associated with chronic hypertension or cardiac valve disease. During anesthesia especially when heart rate increases >115/min or in presence of hypertension or may signal an acute myocardial infarction. It is difficult to diagnose myocardial infarction on ECG in presence of LBBB. The wide QRS complexes characteristic of LBBB may be mistaken for ventricular tachycardia.

Bifascicular Heart Block

Occurs when RBBB + block of one of the fascicles of left bundle branch is present. Most common is RBBB and left anterior hemiblock combination. RBBB + left posterior hemiblock, though uncommon, but progresses to third-degree AV heart block more often.

Insertion of an artificial pacemaker is recommended only when symptomatic bradyarrhythmias occur.

Now, perioperative agents (i.e. change in BP, arterial oxygenation or electrolyte concentrations) might compromise conduction of cardiac impulse in one remaining intact fascicle, leading to sudden onset of third degree AV block.

THIRD-DEGREE AV HEART BLOCK

Characterized by complete absence of the conduction of the cardiac impulse from atria to the ventricles. Continued activity of the ventricles occurrs due to stimulation from an ectopic cardiac pacemaker distal to the site of the conduction block.

If conduction block is near AV node—heart rate is 45-55/min, QRS appears normal. If conduction block is below AV node—heart rate is 30-40/min, QRS complex is wide. Clinical features: Onset is marked by an episode of vertigo and syncope. Syncope associated with seizure is designated as Adams-Stokes attack.

- *Causes*: Primary fibrous degeneration of the conduction system associated with aging (Lenegre's disease), ischemic heart disease, cardiomyopathy, myocarditis, ankylozing spondylitis, iatrogenic after cardiac surgery, congenital (always at the level of AV node), increase in parasympathetic activity, hyperkalemia/other electrolyte derangement.
- *Drugs*: Digitalis, β antagonists and quinidine.
- *Treatment*: Placement of permanent artificial cardiac pacemaker. Prior to which isoproterenol (1-4 μg/min IV) along with atropine may be helpful. Antidysrhythmic drug may suppress the ectopic ventricular pacemaker, so should be avoided.

Events Associated with Initiation of Cardiac Dysrhythmias during Perioperative Period

Arterial hypoxemia, electrolyte disturbances—K, Mg—acid-base imbalance, altered activity of autonomic system, hypertension, intubation of trachea and myocardial ischemia.
- *Drugs*: Catecholamines, volatile anesthetics, co-existing cardiac disease.

Events that Alter Phase 4 (slope) Depolarization

Increase-slope	Decrease slope
Arterial hypoxemia	Vagal stimulation
Hypercarbia	Positive airway pressure
Catecholamines	Acute hyperkalemia
Sympathomimetic drugs	Hypothermia
Acute hypokalemia	
Hyperthermia	
Hypertension	

Disturbances of Cardiac Rhythm (Flowchart 15.7)

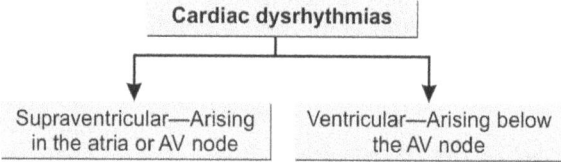

Flowchart 15.7: Disturbances of cardiac rhythm.

Sinus Tachycardia

- *Definition*: Heart rate more than 120/min. It rarely exceeds 200 beats/min.
- *Pathology*: Accelerated discharge rate of SA node.

Causes

- *Preoperative*: Anxiety, pain, sepsis, hypovolemia, fever and CCF.
- *Intraoperative*: Light plane of anesthesia, arterial hypoxemia, hypoglycemia, hyperthyroidism and malignant hyperthermia.
- Sinus tachycardia has a gradual onset and offset. ECG demonstrates P waves with sinus contour proceedings each QRS complex.
- *Treatment*: Sinus tachycardia should not be treated as a primary arrhythmia as it is almost always a physiological response to a demand placed on the heart. Treatment depends on the cause, e.g. digitalis/diuretics for CCF, O_2 for hypoxemia, volume repletion for hypovolemia, etc.

Sinus Bradycardia

- *Definition*: Heart rate less than 60/min due to a deceleration of the normal discharge rate of the SA node.
- *Cause*: Athletic heart syndrome (physiological due to increase in parasympathetic activity), spinal anesthesia, acute diaphragmatic myocardial infarction, halothane, β antagonist administration, hypothermia, jaundice, laryngoscopy, laparoscopy, ECT, traction on ocular muscle/mesentery, drugs like opioids, succinylcholine.
- *Treatment*: IV atropine administration.

Sick Sinus Syndrome (Bradycardia-Tachycardia Syndrome)

It is characterized by bradycardia punctuated by episodes of supraventricular tachycardia most often observed in elderly patient.
- *Pathology*: SA node seems to be vulnerable to exogenous influences.
- *Effects*: Bradycardia may lead to CCF, tachycardia may precipitate angina, systemic embolism in 20% of patients.
- *Treatment*:
  - Placement of artificial cardiac pacemaker, if bradycardia is associated.
  - For tachydysrhythmias: Digitalis, quinidine and β antagonists.
  - For incapacitating tachycardia: Surgical ablation of common bundle and insertion of artificial ventricular pacemaker.

Atrial Premature and Junctional Premature Beats

These arise from ectopic cardiac pacemaker in the atria or near the AV node.

ECG finding: Presence of early and abnormal shaped P waves, but duration of corresponding QRS complex is normal. A distinguishing feature of arterial premature beat is that unlike ventricular premature beat, it is generally not followed by a compensatory pause.

Atrial premature beat can occur in an individual with or without heart disease and is usually insignificant except when it precedes tachydysrhythmias.

Treatment: IV administration of atropine, quinidine is rarely necessary for chronic suppression.

Paroxysmal Supraventricular Tachycardia (PSVT)

Cardiac rhythm of 130-220 beats/min, regular characterized by sudden onset and termination, often initiated by supraventricular premature beat.
- *Pathology*: Functional differences in conduction and refractoriness in the AV node or the presence of AV bypass tract provides for the development of PSVT. Reentry phenomenon is possibly responsible for the development of most of the PSVT.
- *Causes*: WPW syndrome is associated with ASD, Ebstein's anomaly.
- *Effects*: Usually well tolerated, but may precipitate CCF. Polyuria is common.
- *Treatment*: Carotid sinus massage (Application of firm pressure on the carotid sinus, especially the right for 10-20 seconds during constant ECG monitoring). Stimulation of posterior pharynx, perforation of valsalva manicure, electrical cardioversion, adenosine/verapamil also produces conversion.
- *For long-term suppression*: Verapamil, digitalis, β antagonists, quinidine, procainamide are useful.
- OR electrical ablation of AV node with subsequent placement of artificial cardiac pacemaker.

Nonparoxysmal Junctional Tachycardia

- Cardiac rhythm with results from enhanced automaticity or triggered activity in the AV junction.
- *Cause*: Digitalis intoxication (most common), inferior wall myocardial infarction, myocarditis, increased catecholamine, acute rheumatic fever/after effects of cardiac surgery.
- *Treatment*: Stop digitalis—lidocaine/β-blocker, digitalis antibodies (Fab fragments).
- Cardioversion of this rhythm should not be attempted.
- Junctional rhythm leading to decrease in cardiac output and decrease in BP is not infrequent in GA, especially using halothane. IV atropine administration then becomes a necessity.

Atrial Flutter

Characterized on the ECG by an absolutely regular atrial rate of 250–320 beats/min. with varying degrees of AV block often 2:1. The baseline of ECG reveals flutter waves (F waves), resulting in a sawtooth pattern. This dysrhythmia differs from PSVT in that the atrial rate is faster and carotid sinus massage is ineffective/increase in the AV block.

- *Treatment*: Digoxin (0.25–0.75 mg IV) with or without β antagonist or verapamil, electrical cardioversion.

Atrial Fibrillation

Characterized on ECG as totally chaotic atrial activity at a rate of 350–500 beats/min with a corresponding irregular but slower ventricular response. P waves are not discernible on ECG.

- *Causes*
  - Sick sinus syndrome
  - Mitral valvular disease
  - Ischemic heart disease
  - Following thoracic/cardiac surgery
  - Danger of systemic embolization
- *Treatment*: Verapamil (may aggravate CCF), diltiazem (when verapamil is contraindicated), esmolol infusion and anticoagulant therapy.

Ventricular Premature Beats

These arise from a single or multiple ectopic cardiac pacemaker sites located below the AV node.

ECG Findings

- Premature occurrence.
- Absence of a P wave preceding the QRS complex.
- Wide and bizarre-appearing QRS complex.
- ST segment in an opposite direction to QRS complex.
- Inverted T wave.
- Compensatory pause after a premature beat.

Conditions Associated with Appearance of Ventricular Premature Beats (VPB)
- Normal Heart.
- Myocardial hypoxemia, infarction, ischemia.
- Myocarditis.
- Sympathetic overactivity.
- Hypokalemia.
- Hypomagnesemia.
- Digitalis toxicity.
- Central venous/pulmonary A and catheterization.

Treatment

When ventricular premature beats (VPB) are increased 6 beats/min.
- Elimination of the cause.
- Drug of choice is IV lidocaine (1-2 mg/kg IV).
- For chronic suppression—Quinidine, procainamide, disopyramide, amiodarone.

Ventricular Tachycardia
- *Definition*: It is defined as 3/more consecutive ventricular premature beats at a calculated heart rate of greater than 120 beats/min.
- Sustained VT is said to occur when VT persists for > 30 seconds and require termination to prevent hemodynamic collapse.
- *ECG finding*: QRS complexes are widened with no discernible P waves. (rate > 100/min).
- *Causes*: Acute myocardial infarction (common), nonischemic cardiomyopathy, inflammatory/infectious disease of heart, digitalis toxicity.
- Sustained VT produces symptoms due to marked hemodynamic embarrassment but nonsustained VT do not produce symptoms.
- *Result*: May progress to ventricular fibrillation.
- *Treatment*: Prompt electrical cardioversion, IV lidocaine/procainamide (100 mg IV every 2 minutes), bretylium (5 mg/kg IV).

Ventricular Fibrillation
- Characterized by chaotic asynchronous contraction of the ventricles with no visible QRS complexes on ECG.
- There is no effective stroke volume implicating immediate institution of cardiopulmonary resuscitation.
- *Treatment*: Electrical defibrillation is the only effective treatment. In refractory cases, IV lidocaine or bretylium may improve the response to electrical defibrillation.

WOLFF-PARKINSON WHITE SYNDROME (PREEXCITATION SYNDROME)

It is the most common of the preexcitation syndromes, reflecting conduction of the cardiac impulse simultaneously from the SA node down the normal

conduction pathway through AV node and through an accessory pathway (Kent's bundle) that bypasses the AV node.
- *ECG findings*:
  - Short PR interval
  - Wide QRS complex
  - Delta wave.

Wide QRS complex and delta wave reflect the fact that ventricular excitation is a composite of cardiac impulses conducted by a normal and accessory pathway. Delta wave is due to early activation of the ventricle by a cardiac impulse traveling through an accessory pathway.
- *Cause*: Ebstein's anomaly, atrial septal defect (ASD).
- Commonly associated dysrhythmia paroxysmal ventricular tachycardia (PSVT).
- *Result*: Syncope/CCF/both resulting from rapid heart rate. First manifestation may be cardiac arrest and it may appear during the perioperative period.

Management
- Vagal maneuvers, e.g. valsalva, posterior pharynx stimulation.
- Drugs—Verapamil, adenosine, esmolol and procainamide.
- Artificial cardiac pacing.
- Electrical cardioversion.

Special Precautions during Anesthesia
- To avoid sympathetic overactivity.
- Hypovolemia.
- Digoxin.
- Drugs which increase heart rate, e.g. atropine to be avoided. Glycopyrrolate/Scopolamine may be used.
- Ketamine (sympathomimetic effect).
- Pancuronium (has vagolytic effect and increased rate of cardiac impulse).
- Intubation to be done after attaining depth of anesthesia.

LOWN–GANONG–LEVINE SYNDROME

Here conduction occurs through accessory pathways designated as James Fibers, which bypass the AV node and insert directly into the bundle of His. So, normal AV nodal delay is absent.

ECG Findings
- Short PR interval.
- Normal QRS complex.
- Absence of delta wave.

Cardiac dysrhythmias associated: Atrial flutter and atrial fibrillation patients are frequently asymptomatic.
Treatment and management: Same as WPW syndrome.

Mahaim Pathway

Accessory pathway via Mahaim fibers which arise below AV node and insert directly into ventricular muscle.

Adenosine

Antagonist at A_2 receptor (purine) cardiac adenosine receptor type I, peripheral adenosine receptor type 2.

Actions

- Negative inotropic and chronotropic slows conduction via SA and AV node.
- Vascular smooth muscle relaxation → vasodilation.

Duration of action of adenosine is very short 10–20 seconds, patient may feel 'a thump in' the chest.

Uses

- Termination of supraventricular tachycardia (SVT).
- To distinguish supraventricular tachycardia (SVT) from ventricular tachycardia (VT).
- Diagnostic cardiac imaging in patients who cannot exercise.
  To terminate SVT, IV bolus dose of 3 mg/6 mg given; 6 mg repeated after 1–2 hours: then 12 mg (max).
    - *Precautions*: ECG monitoring, continuous cardiac monitoring.
    - *Contraindication*: 2nd/3rd-degree heart block, asthma, atrial flutter (AF), hepatic/renal insufficiency.
    - *Side effects*: Flushing, headache, bronchospasm. If adenosine fails, other drug/DC conversion.

CLASSIFICATION OF ANTIARRHYTHMIC DRUGS

1. Class 1 drugs: Inhibit the fast sodium ion channels.
   Class 1A: Quinidine, procainamide, disopyramide, moricizine
   Class 1B: Lidocaine, tocainide, mexiletine
   Class 1C: Flecainide, propafenone
2. Class II drugs: Decrease the rate of depolarization:
   Propranolol, acebutolol, esmolol
3. Class III drugs: Inhibit potassium ion channels;
   Amiodarone, bretylium, dofetilide, ibutilide, sotalol
4. Class IV drugs: Inhibit slow calcium channels;
   Verapamil, diltiazem.

Efficacy of Antiarrhythmic Drugs in Various Arrhythmias

Drug	Atrial fibrillation	PSVT	Ventricular tachycardia	Remarks
Quinidine	+	++	+	Low therapeutic index
Procainamide	+	++	++	Better tolerated but may cause hypotension
Disopyramide	+	++	++	Anticholinergic side effects; may precipitate CHF
Lidocaine	+	–	++	Used for ventricular arrhythmias
Tocainide	–	–	++	Not in use due to bone marrow suppression
Mexiletine	–	–	++	Orally effective
Moricizine	–	–	++	Reserve drug for ventricular arrhythmias
Flecainide	–	+	++	Useful in VPC, WPW syndrome
Propafenone	–	+	++	May be proarrhythmic
Propranalol	+	++	+	Effective in sympathetic over-activity, torsades de pointes
Amiodarone	+	++	++	Potent drug, can be used preoperatively
Sotalol	++	+	+	Risk of dose-dependent torsades de pointes
Verapamil	+	++	–	Useful in PSVT
Diltiazem	+	++	–	Useful in PSVT only
Digitalis	++	++	–	Used in atrial tachyarrhythmis
Adenosine	–	++	–	Useful in PSVT, WPW syndrome

CHAPTER 16

Anticoagulants, Fibrinolytics and Antiplatelet Agents

INTRODUCTION

Hemostasis is maintained by a delicate balance between coagulation and fibrinolysis so as to maintain normal fluidity of the blood. Thrombi are formed by platelet aggregates, fibrin and trapped RBC. Antiplatelet drugs inhibit platelet aggregation; anticoagulants attenuate fibrin formation while fibrinolytic agents degrade fibrin.

ANTICOAGULANTS

Heparin

Unfractionated heparin is an extract of porcine intestine or bovine lung which are rich in mast cells. It is a polymer of alternating D-glucuronic acid and N-acetyl glucosamine; so it is a sulfated glycosaminoglycan of molecular weight ranging from 3000 to 30,000 daltons.

Mechanism of Action

It acts as an anticoagulant by binding to antithrombin, a circulating serine protease. Heparin enhances the rate of binding of thrombin–antithrombin complex by 1000–10000 times. Other coagulation factors, especially Xa and also XII, XI and IX of the coagulation cascade are also inhibited.

One unit of heparin is defined as the volume of heparin containing solution that will prevent 1 mL of citrated sheep blood from clotting for one hour after addition of 0.2 mL of 1:100 calcium chloride.

Monitoring

Heparin treatment is usually monitored to maintain the ratio of the activated partial prothrombin time (aPTT) within a range of 50–80 seconds. Anti-Xa assay for low-dose regimen should be 0.3–0.5 unit/mL and for high-dose regimen should be 0.5–0.8 unit/mL.

Uses

- Prevention and treatment of deep vein thrombosis and pulmonary embolism.
- Acute coronary syndromes, following myocardial infarction.
- Perioperative anticoagulation for extracorporeal circulation and hemodialysis.

Dosage

Intravenous bolus of 5000–10,000 units followed by continued infusion of 750–1000 units/hr under aPTT monitoring. Deep SC injection of 10,000–20,000 IU every 8–12 hours can also be given if infusion is not possible; intermittent infusion is nowadays not recommended. In low-dose regimen, 5000 IU is given SC every 8–12 hours starting 7–10 days before surgery and continued till the patient is ambulatory (contraindicated in neurosurgery or spinal anesthesia).

Adverse Effects

- Thrombocytopenia—generally mild and transient—can begin within hours of therapy.
- Bleeding due to overdose.
- Osteoporosis on long-term use.
- Hypersensitivity reactions, especially in patients with history of allergic diathesis.

Contraindications of use:
- Bleeding disorders.
- History of heparin-induced thrombocytopenia.
- Severe hypertension.
- Neurosurgery, ocular surgery, lumbar puncture, large malignancies.
- Cirrhosis, renal failure, chronic alcoholics.
- Coadministration of antiplatelet drugs, e.g. Aspirin.

Low Molecular Weight Heparin (LMWH)

Chemical depolymerization of unfractionated heparin yields fragments with mean molecular weight of 4000–5000 daltons. They inhibit factor Xa selectively with little effect on IIa. Therapy with LMWH does not require aPTT monitoring. As route of elimination is primarily by the kidneys, they are contraindicated in renal failure.

Advantages of LMWH Over UFH

- Subcutaneous bioavailability of LMWH is far better than unfractionated heparin (UFH).
- Duration of action is longer, hence once daily administration is enough.
- aPTT monitoring is not necessary.
- Adverse effects like thrombocytopenia or osteoporosis are less frequent.
- Lower incidence of hemorrhagic complications have been reported.

Disadvantages of LMWH

- Cannot be used in cardiopulmonary bypass surgery (less effective in preventing catheter thrombosis).
- Effects are not fully reversed by protamine.

Doses of LMWHs

- Enoxaparin: 20–40 mg OD SC.
- Dalteparin: 200 U/day.
- Reviparin: 0.25 mL SC OD for 7–10 days.
- Parnaparin: 0.6 mL SC OD.
- Ardeparin 2500–5000 IU OD.

Fondaparinux

It is a pentasaccharide with high specificity of binding to antithrombin to inactivate Xa without any effect on IIa; aPTT monitoring is not necessary. Administered subcutaneously, it has a half-life of 15 hours, enabling once daily dosing. It is excreted unchanged by the kidneys, hence contraindicated in renal failure patients. Its bioavailability on SC administration is 100%. Moreover, adverse effects like thrombocytopenia or osteoporosis are least likely to occur. Hence, it is popularly used nowadays.

Idraparinux

Hypermethylated version of fondaparinux with half-life of 80 hours. It can be given once weekly SC It is under phase III trial.

Comparison of Heparin, LMWH and Fondaparinux

Features	Heparin	LMWH	Fondaparinux
Source	Biological	Biological	Synthetic
Molecular weight	15000 daltons	5000 daltons	1500 daltons
Bioavailability	30%	90%	100%
Half-life	1 hour	4 hours	17 hours
Renal excretion	No	Yes	Yes
Target of action	Xa, IIa	Mainly Xa, IIa	Xa only
Antidote action of protamine	Complete	Partial	Absent

Other Parenteral Anticoagulants

- *Lepirudin*: It is a recombinant derivative of hirudin; a direct thrombin inhibitor. It is approved for treatment of patients with heparin-induced thrombocytopenia. It is administered IV under aPTT monitoring. There is no antidote for lepirudin.

- *Desirudin*: Another recombinant derivative of hirudin similar to lepirudin. Chances of hypersensitivity reactions are less.
- *Bivalirudin*: Synthetic analogue of hirudin with half-life of 25 minutes. It is indicated for use in patients with unstable angina undergoing PTCA (percutaneous transluminal coronary angioplasty) and coronary bypass surgery, especially in patients with high risk of heparin-induced thrombocytopenia.
- *Argatroban*: Injectable, synthetic direct thrombin inhibitor indicated for the prophylaxis or treatment of thrombosis in patients with high risk of developing heparin-induced thrombocytopenia. It has the half-life of 40–50 minutes and anticoagulation is reversed after 4 hours of stoppage of drug.

Warfarin

Oral anticoagulant, derivative of 4 hydroxycoumarin is frequently used due to its predictable onset of action, duration of action and excellent bioavailability.

Mechanism of Action

Coagulation factors II, VII, IX, X and anticoagulant proteins C and S are synthesized in the liver but are biologically inactive. The 9-13 amino terminal glutamate residues of the decarboxy precursor protein require reduced vitamin K, catalyzed by γ-glutamyl carboxylase. This carboxylation is coupled to oxidation of vitamin K to its corresponding epoxide. The enzyme responsible for regeneration of active vitamin K is catalyzed by vitamin K epoxide reductase, which is inhibited by warfarin.

Dosage

A dose of 2–5 mg/day for 2–4 days followed by 1–10 mg/day as indicated, under monitoring of INR value with a target of INR 2-3 is appropriate. Lower dose is given to patients with risk of bleeding, including the elderly.

Warfarin is rapidly and completely absorbed orally, intravenously and rectally. It is 97% plasma protein bound leading to a long elimination half life. However, due to the variable half-life of the existing coagulation factors (6-50 hours), onset of action of warfarin is delayed for several days. Warfarin crosses the placental barrier; inactive metabolites are conjugated with glucuronic acid and excreted in bile and urine.

Other Vitamin K Antagonists

Indandione derivatives: Anisindione, phenindione with similar pharmacokinetic profile but with probably a greater incidence of adverse effects.

Phenprocoumon with a longer half-life of about 5 days and slower onset of action compared to warfarin; dose of 0.75-6 mg/day.

Acenocoumarol with the shorter half-life of about 10-24 hours and a shorter duration of action (2 days); dose of 1-8 mg/day.

New Oral Anticoagulants

Dabigatran Etexilate

Prodrug that is converted to dabigatran, which reversibly blocks thrombin; produces a predictable response and monitoring is not necessary. It is approved for prevention of stroke in patients with atrial fibrillation.

Rivaroxaban

Oral drug that inhibits factor Xa. It has 80% bioavailability; given in fixed doses, not require monitoring. It is approved for prophylaxis of venous thromboembolism in patients undergoing hip or knee replacement and also in prevention of stroke in patients with nonvalvular atrial fibrillation.

Apixaban

It is also an orally administered drug, factor Xa inhibitor. It is recommended as 5 mg twice daily in the prevention of stroke and embolism in patients with nonvalvular atrial fibrillation. Dose reduction is necessary in elderly patients, patients with creatinine level >1.5 mg/dL and coadministration with drugs which are hepatic microsomal enzyme inhibitors (e.g. Ketoconazole, itraconazole, clarithromycin) and body weight < 60 kg.

Special precautions to be taken during surgery:
Discontinuation of oral anticoagulant is recommended 1–3 days preoperatively before surgery. Reinstitution of therapy can be done 1–7 days postoperatively, preventing thromboembolic complications in vulnerable patients.

HEPARIN ANTAGONIST (PROTAMINE SULFATE)

Highly basic compound with low molecular weight can be used weight by weight to neutralize heparin. 1 mg is needed to neutralize 100 IU of heparin. Protamine is commonly used when the action of heparin is to be quickly terminated as in cardiac or vascular surgery. It is usually not required as action of heparin disappears within a few hours. It is not effective against fondaparinux and is only partially active against LMWHs. It can release histamine and hypersensitivity reactions have occurred.

The newer oral anticoagulants can increase the incidence of surgical bleeding. For procedures of low hemorrhagic risk, a short window period of 48 hours with drug being stopped 24 hours before surgery and reinstituted after 24 hours of surgery is practiced. For procedures of medium and high risk of bleeding, drug is stopped 5 days prior to surgery and resumed only when risk of bleeding subsides.

PLATELET INHIBITORS

Aspirin

Inhibits cyclooxygenase 1 and TX synthase irreversibly. TXA_2 formation is suppressed till new platelets are formed. Maximal inhibition occurs at low dose (75-150 mg) and prolongation of bleeding time occurs till 7-10 days. Hence, the drug should be stopped 7-10 days before surgical procedure and resumed approximately 24 hours after the surgery.

Dipyridamole

It is a phosphodiesterase inhibitor as well as inhibits uptake of adenosine, thereby increasing cyclic AMP in platelets and inhibits their function. Clinically, the action of dipyridamole is insignificant. It enhances the action of warfarin or aspirin when administered together.

Clopidogrel

Thienopyridine, which selectively and irreversibly blocks $P2Y_{12}$ and inhibits the binding of ADP, thereby inhibiting platelet function. It is a prodrug with 50% bioavailability, potent, onset of action takes about 4 hours but action lasts for 5-7 days. Dose is 75 mg OD. Adverse effects are diarrhea, epigastric pain and skin rashes.

Ticlopidine

Thienopyridine which inhibits ADP, irreversibly block $P2Y_{12}$, fibrinogen binding to platelets is prevented. As there is no effect on platelet TXA_2, it is synergistic in action to aspirin. The drug is well absorbed orally, peak effect is produced after 8-10 days and lasts for 5-6 days. Serious adverse effects like thrombocytopenia, neutropenia and hemolysis have made it unpopular.

Prasugrel

Most potent and fast-acting $P2Y_{12}$ receptor blocker. It is a prodrug, rapidly absorbed and rapidly activated, particularly useful in acute coronary syndromes, STEMI but is contraindicated in patients with risk of intracranial hemorrhage. Dose is 5-10 mg OD.

Abciximab

It is Fab fragment of a chimeric monoclonal Ab, active against GP II_b/III_a protein. After a bolus dose, platelet aggregation remains inhibited for 12-24 hours. After a bolus dose, especially in acute coronary syndrome, platelet remains inhibited for 12-24 hours. Dose is 0.25 mg/kg IV 10-60 min before PCI. Adverse effect is hemorrhage and thrombocytopenia.

ASRA Practice Advisory Anticoagulation, 3rd edition, 2010, recommend the following:
- Clopidogrel should be discontinued for 7 days prior to performing neuraxial block.
- Enoxaparin to be stopped for 10-12 hours before neuraxial needle placement.
- Enoxaparin can be started only after 2 hours of epidural catheter removal.
- Epidural catheter should only be removed, if INR is below 1.5.

FIBRINOLYTICS

These drugs are used to lyse clots occluding blood vessels and acts primarily by generation of plasmin. The major aim of thrombolysis is to achieve reperfusion and prevent mortality, especially when major coronary artery is involved. Venous thrombi are lysed more easily than arterial thrombi and these fibrinolytics are of minimum therapeutic use in clots more than 3 days old. The fibrinolytics commonly used are; streptokinase, urokinase, alteplase, reteplase, tenecteplase.

Streptokinase

Derived from β hemolytic streptococci group C, was the first fibrinolytic to be used. Streptokinase after activation on combination with circulating plasminogen, acted upon the rest of plasminogen to produce plasmin, which caused clot lysis. It has now come to disuse due to its decreased efficacy as a result of antistreptococcal antibodies, greater chance of adverse effects like hypersensitivity and bleeding, also less specificity compared to the newer agents available now.

Urokinase

The enzyme derived from human urine, hence the name was commercially prepared and used in patients antigenic to streptokinase. Though it is non-antigenic with lesser incidence of side effects, it is also seldom used now.

Alteplase

Recombinant tissue plasminogen activator, acts on fibrin bound plasminogen, is nonantigenic with short half-life of 4-8 minutes. Hence, it is given by IV bolus of 50 mg administered over 30 minute followed by 35 mg over 1 hour, in myocardial infarction and 100 mg over 2 hours in pulmonary embolism, followed by slow infusion of 0.9 mg/kg/hr.

Reteplase

It is a mutant of alteplase with longer duration of action. Dose 10 mg over 10 min repeated after 30 min.

Tenecteplase

Genetically engineered mutant of native tPA, has longer duration of action, decreased plasma clearance and more specificity of action. Dose 0.5 mg/kg single bolus injection.

Indications of Use

- Acute myocardial infarction.
- Pulmonary embolism.
- Peripheral arterial occlusion.
- Stroke.
- Deep vein thrombosis.

Contraindications of Use
- History of bleeding diathesis.
- History of stroke, head injury within last 3 months.
- History of major surgery within last 3 weeks.
- Bleeding peptic ulcer or bleeding varices.
- Pregnancy.
- Vascular anomalies or aneurysms.
- Uncontrolled hypertension.

CHAPTER 17

Drugs Used in Central Nervous System

DRUGS USED IN PARKINSONISM

LEVODOPA

- L-3, 4-dihydroxyphenylalanine, the metabolic precursor of dopamine (DA).
- Rapidly absorbed orally from small intestine by transport system of amino acids.
- Concentration of the drug in plasma peaks in 0.5–2 hours after an oral dose.
- Half-life is 1–3 hours.
- Rate and extent of absorption of levodopa depends on the rate of gastric emptying, pH of gastric juice, time of exposure to degenerative enzyme of gastric and intestinal mucosa and presence of amino acids in diet.
- Entry of the drug into central nervous system (CNS) across the blood-brain barrier (BBB) is mediated by membrane transporter for aromatic amino acids.
- Levodopa is converted to DA by decarboxylation in the presynaptic terminals of dopaminergic neurons in the striatum.
- This dopamine is available for therapeutic action.
- After release, it is either transported back to dopaminergic terminals by uptake mechanism or metabolized by monoamine oxidase (MAO) or catechol-o-methyltransferase (COMT).
- In clinical practice, levodopa is always administered in combination with peripherally acting inhibitor of aromatic L-amino acid decarboxylase, e.g. carbidopa or benserazide.
- If levodopa is administered alone, the drug is largely decarboxylated by enzymes in the intestinal mucosa and peripheral sites, such that < 1% of levodopa can ultimately cross the blood brain barrier.
- 25 mg of carbidopa and 100 mg of levodopa combination given 3 times or more daily.

- Levodopa produces dramatic improvement in early phase of disease but with time, its buffering capacity is lost with onset of motor complications like disabling dyskinesias.

Adverse Effects of Levodopa

- Nausea, motor complications, hallucinations, confusion occur, especially in elderly (clozapine and quetiapine appear to be effective).
- Activation of vascular DA receptors may produce orthostatic hypotension.
- *'Wearing off' phenomenon*: Each dose of levodopa being effective only for a period of 1-2 hours; with reappearance of symptoms. Increase in dose and frequency can benefit to some extent but will result in:
  - Dyskinesia: Excessive and abnormal involuntary movements especially when plasma concentration of levodopa is high.
  - 'On-off' phenomenon, waxing and waning of symptoms.
  - Abrupt withdrawal of levodopa or other dopaminergic medications may precipitate 'neuroleptic malignant syndrome' of confusion, rigidity and hyperthermia and may be potentially lethal.

DOPAMINE RECEPTOR AGONISTS

- Direct agonists of striatal DA receptors.
- Enzymatic conversion is not required for necessary activity; hence does not depend on functional capacities of nigrostriatal neurons.
- Longer duration of action compared to levodopa.
- Often used in the management of dose-related fluctuations of motor state.
- May modify the course of PD by reducing endogenous release of DA, need of exogenous L-dopa and decrease in formation of free radical.
- Ropinirole and pramipexole are better tolerated than older agents, bromocriptine and pergolide.
- Selective activity at D_2 and D_3 receptors, no action on D_1 family.
- Absorbed orally, relieve symptoms of parkinsonism disease (PD) (like dopa).
- *Side effects*: Hallucinosis, confusion, nausea, orthostatic hypotension, fatigue and somnolence.
- Initiated at low dose and titrated slowly.
- It is better to switch over to some other agent if somnolence is troublesome.

Apomorphine

- Dopaminergic agonist administered SC.
- It has been used as 'rescue therapy' in management of 'on-off' phenomenon' of L-dopa therapy.
- Highly emetogenic, side effects similar to other DA agonists.
- Concomitant use of apomorphine and $5HT_3$ antagonist like ondansetron is contraindicated (C/I) due to profound hypotension and loss of consciousness.

- It has high affinity to D_4 with moderate affinity to D_2, D_3 and D_5 receptors, low affinity to D_1 receptors. It also has moderate affinity to α_{1D}, α_{2B} and α_{2C} receptors.
- Apomorphine therapy should be initiated with a 2 mg test dose in a setting where the patient can be monitored carefully.

COMT INHIBITORS

- Principal therapeutic action of catechol-o-methyltransferase (COMT) inhibitor is to block the peripheral conversion of levodopa to 3-o-methyl DOPA, increasing both plasma t½ of levodopa and fraction of levodopa (each dose) which reaches CNS.
- The COMT inhibitors tolcapone and entacapone differ only in pharmacokinetic activities and adverse effects.
- Tolcapone has longer duration of action and appears to inhibit both peripheral and central COMT.
- Entacapone has a shorter duration of action and principally inhibits peripheral COMT.
- Common adverse effects are nausea, orthostatic hypotension, confusion and hallucination.
- Important adverse effects of tolcapone is hepatotoxicity; fatal fulminant hepatic failure has been reported.

SELECTIVE MAO INHIBITORS

- The isoenzyme MAO-B is the predominant form in the striatum and responsible for most of the oxidative metabolism of dopamine (DA) in brain.
- Two selective MAO-B inhibitors commonly used are selegiline and rasagiline.
- Produce modest beneficial effects on symptoms of Parkinson's disease (PD).
- Selegiline has been used for years and tolerated well in younger patients with early or mild disease.
- In advanced stage, selegiline may accentuate the adverse motor and cognitive effects of levodopa therapy.
- Recently, orally disintegrating tablet or transdermal patch of selegiline is being used to prevent first pass metabolism and formation of amphetamine metabolites.
- Rasagiline does not produce amphetamine metabolites; effective as monotherapy in early PD, significantly reducing levodopa-related 'wearing off' symptoms.
- Rasagiline may have a neuroprotective role.
- MAO-B inhibitors are well-tolerated but drug interactions are troublesome.

MUSCARINIC RECEPTOR ANTAGONISTS

- Trihexyphenidyl (2-4 mg TDS) and benztropine (1-4 mg BD) are currently used in the treatment of drug-induced parkinsonism.
- Diphenhydramine also with antihistaminic action can also be used.
- All are adjunct drugs to dopaminergic therapy.
- *Side effects*: Sedation, mental confusion, constipation, urinary retention and blurred vision are other adverse effects.

Amantadine

- Antiviral drug against influenza A, appears to alter DA release in striatum.
- It also has anticholinergic activity and blocks NMDA glutamate receptors.
- Its action is modest, hence used as initial treatment mild PD.
- *100 mg BD; Side effects*: Dizziness, lethargy, sleep disturbance, anticholinergic effects, nausea and vomiting.

Summary

- Levodopa and carbidopa combination is drug of choice as therapy.
- Dopamine receptor agonists may be used as sole therapy initially or when L-DOPA fails to produce effect.
- Anticholinergics are preferred in young patients, where tremor is the main symptom.
- Drugs in general may be grouped as symptomatic therapy and neuroprotective therapy.
- Dopamine agonists and rasagiline have neuroprotective role.
    - Endogenous and exogenous catecholamines are metabolized mainly by two enzymes MAO and COMT. MAO occurs within cells bound to the surface membrane of mitochondria.
    - MAO is abundant in NA neurons and other tissues like liver and intestinal epithelium.
    - MAO converts catecholamines to their corresponding aldehydes; yields DOMA from NA.
    - MAO oxidizes other monoamines, e.g. dopamine and 5HT.

DRUG-INDUCED PARKINSONISM

Chlorpromazine acts on all dopaminergic receptors but especially on D_2, D_3 receptors. Dopamine activity as well as release are affected. Decrease in dopaminergic activity results in drug-induced parkinsonism, associated with tremor, rigidity and bradykinesia.

Treatment is started with a low dose of one of the centrally acting anticholinergic drugs. These drugs can improve the tremor and rigidity of parkinsonism but has little effect on bradykinesia. They have higher central peripheral anticholinergic action.

Drugs Given
- Benztropine mesylate 1-6 mg/day.
- Biperiden 2-12 mg/day.
- Orphenadrine 150-400 mg/day.
- Procyclidine 75-30 mg/day.
- Trihexyphenidyl 6-20 mg/day.

Action
Acts by decreasing the unbalanced cholinergic activity.

Side Effects
- *CNS effects*: Drowsiness, mental slowness, inattention, restlessness, confusion, agitation, delusions, hallucinations and mood changes.
- *Other effects*: Dryness of mouth, blurring of vision, urinary retention, constipation, tachycardia, tachypnea and increase in IOT.
- *Contraindications*: Prostatic hyperplasia, obstructive GI disease, e.g. pyloric stenosis angle closure glaucoma.
- If medication has to be withdrawn, this should be accomplished gradually rather than abruptly in order to prevent acute exacerbation of parkinsonism.
- *Drug interaction*: Following drugs should not be used concurrently, e.g. TCA, antihistaminics because they can precipitate complications.
- The traditional antipsychotics bind D_2 receptor 50 times more avidly than D_1 or D_3 receptors—this D_2 antagonism is responsible for EPS side effect.

Distribution of Dopamine Receptors
- *Cortex*: Responsible for arousal and mood.
- *Limbic system*: Emotion and stereotypical behavior.
- *Striatum*: Motor control.
- *Ventral hypothalamus and anterior pituitary*: Prolactin secretion.

Drugs causing EPS
Extrapyramidal syndrome (EPS), particularly prominent with high potency D_2 dopamine receptor antagonists, e.g. Tricyclic piperazines and butyrophenones and less likely with aripiprazole, clozapine quetiapine or risperidone.

Time of onset: 5-30 days but can occur even after a single dose.

ANTIDEPRESSANTS

INTRODUCTION

Depression and anxiety disorders involve variations in mood, behavior cognition and somatic function and are amenable to pharmacological treatment. Depressive episodes are characterized by sadness, pessimism, lack of concentration, insomnia, mental slowing, feeling of guilt and worthlessness.

Antidepressants used are as follows (Table 17.1):
- *Selective serotonin reuptake inhibitors (SSRIs)*: Sertraline, fluoxetine, fluvoxamine, citalopram, escitalopram and paroxetine.
- *Selective serotonin and norepinephrine reuptake inhibitors (SNRIs)*: Venlafaxine, duloxetine and desvenlafaxine.
- *Atypical antidepressants (5HT$_2$ receptor antagonists)*: Duloxetine, mirtazapine, mianserin, bupropion, nefazodone and trazodone.

Table 17.1: Mechanism of action of antidepressants.

Drug	Action	Adverse effects	Use
Trazodone	Weakly blocks 5HT uptake, weak 5HT$_2$ antagonistic activity, α_1 adrenergic blocking action	Sedation, bradycardia, postural hypotension, priapism	Major depression
Mirtazapine	Blocks α_2 auto and hetero-receptors, increases both NA and 5HT release concurrent block of 5HT$_2$, 5HT$_3$ receptors, additional H$_1$ receptor blockade	Sedation, increase in appetite, weight gain, rarely agranulocytosis	Do
Mianserin	Blocks presynaptic α_2 receptors, increase in NA antagonistic action on 5HT$_2$, 5HT$_1$ and H$_1$ receptors	Sedation, anxiolysis, seizure, liver dysfunction, blood dyscrasia	Depression with anxiety
Bupropion	Inhibitor of NA and dopamine non-sedative antidepressant, prolonged elimination, half-life 11 hours	Agitation, insomnia, dry mouth, seizures in high dose	Smoking cessation
Tianeptine	Increase in 5HT uptake but has antidepressant and antianxiolytic effect	Insomnia/drowsiness, dry mouth, body-ache, tremor	Depression with anxiety
Amineptine	Increase in 5HT uptake but has antidepressant activity	Anticholinergic side effects, e.g. tachycardia, dry mouth, CVS side effects, e.g. postural hypotension, arrhythmias	Do

- *Tricyclic antidepressants*:
  - Amitriptyline
  - Clomipramine
  - Imipramine
  - Doxepin
  - Amoxapine
  - Nortriphyline
  - Protriptyline
  - Maprotiline
- *Monoamine oxidase inhibitors*:
  - MAO-A inhibitor: Moclobemide
  - MAO-B inhibitor: Selegiline.

MECHANISM OF ACTION

The reuptake inhibitors increase the respective neurotransmitter levels by inhibiting the transporters; SERT (serotonin transporter) or NET (norepinephrine transporter) or both. Tricyclic antidepressants increase 5HT and NE level by inhibiting their reuptake while the monoamine oxidase (MAO) acts by inhibiting the metabolism of monoamine neurotransmitters, 5HT, NE and or dopamine. MAO-A and MAO-B are involved in metabolizing both 5HT and NE and are present in mitochondria of most neurons. MAO-B is present in serotonergic neurons.

LONG-TERM EFFECTS OF ANTIDEPRESSANTS

- Increase in adrenergic and serotonergic receptors.
- Increased receptor functioning.
- Increase in neurotropic factors.
- Increase in neurogenesis.

There is usually a period of 'therapeutic lag' of about 3-4 weeks, before antidepressant action becomes evident. After successful initiation of therapy, a maintenance therapy of 6-12 months is generally necessary after which the drug is gradually tapered off. Major depression of > 2 years duration often requires life-long therapy.

1. **Selective serotonin reuptake inhibitors (SSRIs):** Clinically used SSRIs are relatively selective in inhibiting SERT compared to NET and increase as well as prolong serotonergic neurotransmission. They do not have action on histaminic, muscarinic or other receptors.
   - Plasma half-life about 22-33 hours, with fluoxetine having longest half-life (48-72 hours).
   - Plasma protein binding 80-98%.
   - Potent inhibitors of CYP2D6 resulting in drug interactions (fluoxetine, paroxetine) fluvoxamine, inhibitor of CYP3A4 while citalopram, escitalopram and sertraline have few drug interactions.
   - Relatively safe drugs with minimum adverse effects.
   - They are devoid of cardiovascular, anticholinergic or neurological side effects.
   - Main adverse effects are gastrointestinal (GI) and sexual dysfunction.
   - *Indication for use*: Major depression, anxiety, panic disorders, post-traumatic stress disorder, obsessive-compulsive disorder, postmenopausal dysphoric symptoms.

2. **Tricyclic antidepressants:** The tricyclic antidepressants or tertiary amine tricyclics act by increasing both 5HT and NE inhibiting their reuptake. They have become unpopular due to their adverse effects and chance of lethality due to overdose. They are used only when other antidepressants are not effective.
   - Act primarily by increasing NE and 5HT. Also act on H_1, $5HT_2$, α_1 and muscarinic receptors.
   - Potent anticholinergic action causing dry mouth, blurred vision, constipation and urinary retention.
   - Postural hypotension due to α_1 blockade, cardiac arrhythmias with ECG changes are seen.
   - Central nervous system (CNS) effects like sedation, lack of concentration, lethargy, convulsions may occur. Weight gain creates a problem.
   - Well-absorbed orally.
   - Long plasma half-life so once daily dosing.
   - Metabolized by CYP2D6, CYP3A4 or CYP1A2 leading to drug interactions.
   - Relatively narrow therapeutic window; plasma concentration monitoring may be necessary.
   - *Uses*: Depression, unresponsive to other medications, various types of pain, enuresis and insomnia.
   - *Drug interactions*: Should not be combined with SSRI or monoamine oxidase inhibitors (MAOIs) dangerous toxicity can occur. TCAs decrease the action of indirectly acting sympathomimetics, antihypertensives like guanethidine, clonidine TCAs potentiate CNS depressants. The secondary amine tricyclics which selectively increase NE levels have actions similar to but lesser extent of adverse effects compared to the tertiary amine tricyclics. Adverse effects like sedation, anticholinergic action or weight gain are comparatively less.

   One tricyclic antidepressant (TCA), amoxapine has additional dopamine receptor antagonistic action and has extrapyramidal syndrome (EPS) adverse effects like tardive dyskinesia.

3. **Serotonin and norepinephrine reuptake inhibitors (SNRIs):**
   - All SNRIs bind to serotonin and NE transporters but unlike the TCAs, they do not bind to other receptors.
   - Plasma half-life of 11–12 hours; once daily dosing.
   - Minimum plasma protein binding except duloxetine, which undergoes extensive hepatic metabolism.
   - *Side effects*: Better tolerability, side effect profile similar to that of SSRIs like nausea, constipation, headache, insomnia and sexual dysfunction. Venlafaxine may cause sustained diastolic hypertension, hence available in extended release form.
   - *Use*: Favored over TCAs for treatment of major depression and pain syndromes.

4. **Atypical antidepressants:** Most of these drugs are antagonists of $5HT_2$ group of receptors and have antidepressant activity. They are often given

in combination with SSRIs. Though blockade of $5HT_{2A}$ receptor is most marked, they have affinity towards other 5HT receptors or α receptor or H_1 receptor as well. So, their mechanism of action is atypical compared to other antidepressants.

5. **Monoamine oxidase inhibitors:**
   - These are rarely used due to their major food and drug interactions and toxicities.
   - Irreversible inhibition of MAO-A and MAO-B leads to increase of endogenous monoamines like 5HT, NA and dopamine resulting in various adverse effects and exogenous monoamines like tyramine in food.
   - Interacts with other antidepressants like SSRIs, SNRIs, and TCAs to cause serotonin syndrome.

Points to note:
Excess stimulation of 5HT receptors results in the following effects:
- *CNS*: Delirium, coma and tremor.
- *CVS*: Tachycardia, hypertension and diaphoresis.
- *Somatic*: Hyperreflexia and myoclonus.

All serotonergic drugs should be withdrawn for at least 2 weeks before starting an MAOI; for fluoxetine, the withdrawal period should be 4–5 weeks. Similarly, MAOI should be discontinued for at least 2 weeks before starting any serotonergic agent.

- When MAOIs are given in addition to tyramine in diet; the patients may suffer from malignant hypertension or myocardial infarction or stroke; also known as 'cheese reaction'. So patients on MAOIs should avoid foods like aged cheeses, tap beer, soy products, dried sausages and require a low-tyramine diet.
- Monoamine oxidase inhibitors (MAOIs), which inhibit both MAO-A and MAO-B are tranylcypromine, phenelzine and isocarboxazid. MAO-A inhibitor moclobemide and MAO-B inhibitor selegiline are rather used.
- To avoid high first pass metabolism, selegiline is available as transdermal patch or sublingual forms to increase BA.

Precautions to be Maintained during Anesthesia:
- There are chances of dangerous drug interactions in patients on MAO inhibitors. Sympathomimetic drugs may precipitate potentially dangerous hypertensive crises.
- Opioid drugs like pethidine, tramadol and dextromethorphan, which have serotonergic properties, may precipitate serotonin syndrome.
- MAO inhibitors can inhibit hepatic microsomal enzymes and increase the serum concentration of opioids, enhancing chances of toxicity.
- Pancuronium should be avoided in these patients as it releases stored NA.
- Phenelzine can decrease plasma cholinesterase level, thereby increasing the duration of action of succinylcholine.
- Use of cocaine should be prevented, other local anesthetics (LAs) are safe.

- Among the opioids, morphine can be safely used, though fentanyl, alfentanil, sufentanil or remifentanil are not contraindicated.
- Of the vasopressor agents, felypressin is used instead of adrenaline.
- If patient is on antipsychotic drug, it should not be abruptly withdrawn.
- Antipsychotic drugs may potentiate the sedative and hypotensive actions of anesthetic agents.
- Lithium potentiates both depolarizing and nondepolarizing muscle relaxants.
- Nonsteroidal anti-inflammatory drugs (NSAIDs) should preferably not be used in patients on lithium.

ANESTHETIC IMPLICATIONS IN PATIENTS ON ANTIEPILEPTIC DRUGS

Epilepsy is a disorder associated with abnormal discharges in brain followed by unpredictable episodes of seizures, loss or altered consciousness and need prolonged therapy of antiepileptic drugs.
- Preanesthetic medication with sedatives like benzodiazepines, e.g. lorazepam/diazepam is essential.
- Thiopentone is preferred as inducing agent.
- Muscle relaxants without a steroid nucleus, e.g. atracurium or cisatracurium are safe (phenytoin causes rapid metabolism of vecuronium/rocuronium).
- Local anesthetics can be administered within safety limit under close monitoring.
- Of the antiemetics, metoclopramide should be avoided. Ondansetron or domperidone to be used instead.

Precautions regarding use of the following drugs:
- Ketamine.
- Methohexital.
- Propofol.
- Etomidate.
- Enflurane.
- Antiemetics: Metoclopramide, droperidol and phenothiazines.
- Muscle relaxants: Vecuronium and rocuronium.

Point to note: Most of the commonly used antiepileptics are inducers of microsomal enzymes which lead to various drug interactions. Plasma concentration of antiepileptics need to be monitored in the perioperative period to avoid complications.

CHAPTER 18

Drugs Acting on Endocrine System

ANTIDIABETIC DRUGS

PREOPERATIVE GLYCEMIC GOALS

Fasting blood sugar level 90–130 mg/dL, postprandial blood sugar level <180 mg/dL, HbA1c level <7% and currently ADA recommends that blood glucose level should be maintained between 140 mg/dL and 180 mg/dL in critically ill patients.

INSULIN IN TREATMENT OF DIABETES

Insulin Types

- Porcine and bovine insulins have now been replaced by recombinant human insulins:
  - *Short-acting*: Regular/soluble insulin onset in 15–30 minutes lasts for 5–7 hours.
  - *Intermediate*: Insulin zinc suspension (lente). Mixture of 30% short acting and 70% ultralente insulin.
    Onset 2–4 hours, peak duration 18–24 hours.
    Neutral protamine Hagedorn (NPH) or isophane insulin.
    2 parts soluble crystalline zinc insulin, 1 part protamine zinc insulin.
  - *Long-acting*: Ultralente or relatively insoluble protamine zinc-insulin suspension in an acetate buffer. Onset of action quite delayed, up to 36 hours.
  - *Insulin analogs*: Newer insulins;
    Rapid-acting—(i) Insulin lispro (ii) insulin aspart and (iii) insulin glulysine
    long-acting—(i) insulin glargine and (ii) insulin determir.
  - *Insulin mixtures*: 70% NPH + 30% regular.
    50% NPH + 50% regular.
    The NPH preparation does not contain excess protamine, does not delay absorption, preferred over lente.
- Insulin lispro or insulin glargine is not FDA approved for use in pregnancy.

METHODS OF INSULIN THERAPY

Intensive therapy: Total insulin requirement is:
- *Weight of patient in pounds* divided by 4 = Units of insulin required/day.
- *0.55 × body weight (kg)* = Units of insulin required/day.

Half of the total requirement should provide the basal requirement while the rest divided for treating postmeal hyperglycemia. However, dose requirement should be individualized.

Typical total daily basal dose of insulin: body weight (kg) × 0.3. IU of insulin, decrease blood sugar level by 50 mg/dL.

Conventional therapy: Also known as sliding scale regimen, where intermediate or long-acting dose is fixed while short or rapid insulin dose varies according to blood glucose level.

Insulin Delivery Devices

- Jet injector system.
- Single unit syringe.
- Portable pen injectors with cartridge containing 100 µ.
- Continuous subcutaneous infusion of insulin (CSII) through computerized pump.
- Intraperitoneal delivery device.
- Implantable pellets SC.
- Closed loop artificial pancreas.
- Oral, nasal and rectal.
- Inhalational—achieved by addition of various adjuvants, e.g. mannitol, glycine and sodium citrate.
- Transplantation or gene therapy.

DIABETIC KETOACIDOSIS

Life-threatening medical emergency occurring in type 1 DM patients occasionally in type 2 DM patients associated with nausea, vomiting, abdominal pain, altered mental status, hyperglycemia and ketoacidosis. Treatment;
- Rehydration with NS followed by ½ NS, then DNS.
- Maintenance of K and other electrolyte balance monitored by serum level and ECG changes; KCl 10–20 mEq/hr if required.
- Regular human insulin in bolus dose of 0.1–0.2 U/kg IV followed by 0.1 U/kg/hr till hyperglycemia is controlled.
- $NaHCO_3$ 50 mEq to be added to IV fluid if blood pH less than 7.1.

HYPEROSMOLAR NONKETOTIC COMA

It occurs in type 2 DM patients, associated with high blood glucose, more than 600 mg/dL; high blood osmolality, with blood glucose >800 mg/dL resulting in plasma osmolality > 350 mOsm/L leads to coma.

- *Treatment*: Aggressive rehydration, electrolyte homeostasis and insulin therapy at the rate of 0.1 U/kg/hr.

HYPOGLYCEMIA

- Often associated complication of insulin therapy.
- S/S-marked autonomic overactivity, e.g. tachycardia, palpitation, sweating, tremor, nausea; may progress to convulsion and coma.
- *Treatment*: If patient is conscious, simple sugar like glucose orally preferably in liquid form. Dextrose tablets, glucose gel or sugar containing beverage or food can be given. If patient is unconscious;
  - 20–50 mL of 50% glucose iv over 2–3 minutes as IV infusion, or
  - 1 mg glucagon SC.

Complications of Insulin Therapy

- Hypoglycemia.
- Insulin allergy.
- Insulin resistance.
- Lipodystrophy at injection site.
- Short-lived dependent edema due to salt retention.

Drug Interactions

- Drugs which increase blood sugar level and may cause insulin resistance:
  - Thiazides and furosemide
  - OCPs
  - Corticosteroids
  - Salbutamol
  - Nifedipine.
- Drugs which decrease blood sugar and may induce hypoglycemia:
  - Acute ingestion of alcohol
  - Lithium
  - Beta blockers
  - High dose aspirin therapy
  - Theophylline.

ORAL ANTIDIABETIC AGENTS

Classification (Table 18.1)

- *Sulfonylureas*: First generation—tolbutamide and tolazamide.
  Second generation: Glimeperide, glibenclamide, glipizide and gliclazide.
- *Biguanide*: Metformin.
- *Meglitinides*: Rapaglinide and nateglinide.
- *Thiazolidinediones*: Rosiglitazone and pioglitazone.
- *Alpha glucosidase inhibitors*: Acarbose, miglitol and voglibose.
- *GLP-1 agonists*: Exenatide and liraglutide (injectables).
- *Dipeptidyl peptidase*: 4 inhibitors—sitagliptin, vildagliptin and saxagliptin.

Table 18.1: Comparative study of various antidiabetic agents.

Drug	Duration	Dose/day	Indications	Adverse effects
Glimeperide Glibenclaminde Glipizide Gliclazide	24 hr 24 hr 12 hr 12–24 hr	1–6 mg OD/BD 2.5–15 mg OD/BD 5–20 mg BD 40–240 mg OD/BD	1st line therapy in type 2 DM	Hypoglycemia Weight gain
Metformin	6–8 hr	500 mg–2.5 g BD	1st line/add on drug in type 2 DM	Anorexia, nausea, weight reduction
Pioglitazone	24 hr	15–30 mg OD/BD	1st line/add on drug	Edema, weight gain
Repaglinide Nateglinide	3–5 hr 2–4 hr	1–8 mg BD/TDS 180–480 mg TDS	Postprandial hyperglycemia	Hypoglycemia, Nausea, Jt pain
Acarbose miglitol voglibose		50–100 mg TDS 25–100 mg TDS 200–300 mg TDS	Postprandial hyperglycemia	GI discomfort, flatulence, diarrhea
Sitagliptin Vildagliptin Saxagliptin	12–16 hr 12–24 hr 24 hr	100 mg BD 50–100 mg BD 2.5–5 mg OD	Add on drug in type 2 DM	Rhinitis, URTI, headache, pancreatitis
Pramlintide	2–3 hr	Given SC as inj	Types 1 and 2 DM	Nausea, anorexia
Exenatide Liraglutide	6–10 hr 24 hr	Given SC as inj	As add on drug in type 2 DM	Nausea, anorexia, mild weight loss, pancreatitis
Colesevelam hydrochloride	24 hr	625 mg tablet, 3 tablets BD	Type 2 DM	Constipation, indigestion

- *Sodium glucose cotransporter*: 2 inhibitor—dapagliflozin.
- *Amylin analog*: Pramlintide.
- *Bile acid sequestrants*: Colesevelam.

Mechanism of Action

Sulfonylureas and meglitinides are **insulin secretagogues** while metformin and pioglitazone are considered to reduce insulin resistance and are called **insulin sensitizers**. The alpha glucosidase inhibitors inhibit alpha glucosidases of gut and interferes with carbohydrate degradation and absorption. Sitagliptin is a selective **DPP-4 inhibitor** while saxagliptin and vildagliptin bind to DPP-4 covalently and **potentiates the action of GLP-1** and **GIP**, which increase postprandial insulin secretion. GLP-1 receptor agonists exenatide, liraglutide induce insulin secretion while amylin analog, pramlintide acts centrally to induce early satiety. SGLT-2 inhibitor, dapagliflozin, causes **glycosuria** and decreases blood sugar level. Colesevelam probably **decreases glucose absorption from gut**, mechanism of action has not yet been established.

Preoperative and Perioperative Steps for the Diabetic Patient

Preoperative Preparation

- If the patient is on insulin NPH/regular, 2/3rd of insulin dose taken to be administered the night before and half the usual dose in the morning. If on insulin pump; it should be decreased to 30%. If on glargine and lispro/aspart, morning dose is to be omitted. Oral antidiabetics are to be discontinued 24-48 hours before OT. Intraoperative blood glucose should be within 120–180 mg/dL.
- Stop oral antidiabetic drugs 24 hours before surgery.
- Type 1 diabetes patients should not go without insulin.
- Blood glucose level should be maintained between 4 and 10 mmol/L.
- Fast from midnight onward, blood glucose maintained by insulin/glucose drip.
- Insulin therapy to be decided depending upon blood glucose level. Blood potassium level should also be monitored and KCl to be added to each 500 mL of 5% dextrose bottle accordingly given in Tables 18.2 and 18.3.

Table 18.2: Blood glucose level monitoring.

Blood glucose level (mmol/L)	Soluble insulin to be added in 500 mL of 5% dextrose
<4 mmol/L	5 U
4–6 mmol/L	10 U
6.1–10 mmol/L	15 U
10.1–20 mmol/L	20 U

Table 18.3: Blood potassium level monitoring.

Blood potassium level	KCl to be added to each 500 mL of 5% dextrose
<3 mmol/L	20 mmol
3–5 mmol/L	10 mmol
≥5 mmol/L	Not required

DRUGS USED IN THYROID DISORDERS

- The hypothyroid patient is treated with L-thyroxine sodium 25/50/100 µg tablet daily at breakfast. Therapy should be started at minimum dose required and increased gradually over weeks until the patient becomes euthyroid, when maintenance therapy is continued.
- Liothyronine/triiodothyronine can be occasionally used along with L-thyroxine in myxedema coma but it is not easily available. Clinically however, L-thyroxine is preferred for its uniform, sustained action and less propensity of cardiac arrhythmias.

ANTITHYROID DRUGS

Drugs which interfere with the synthesis of thyroid hormones. The antithyroid drugs that have clinical utility are:
- *Thioamides*: Methimazole, carbimazole, propylthiouracil.
- Iodides.
- Radioactive Iodine.

Mechanism of Action

- Inhibit the incorporation of iodine into tyrosyl residues of thyroglobulin.
- Also inhibit the coupling of these iodotyrosyl residues to form iodothyronine.
- Bind to and inactivate the peroxidase only when the heme of the enzyme is in oxidized state.

The coupling reaction is more sensitive to antithyroid drug, such as propylthiouracil. In addition to blocking hormone synthesis, propylthiouracil partially inhibits the peripheral deiodination of T4 to T3.

Pharmacodynamics

Propylthiouracil is 75% protein bound and plasma ½ life 75 minutes; carbimazole/methimazole are less protein bound and greater ½ life. The latter are more potent and require once daily dosing; quickly absorbed orally, widely distributed in the body.

Side Effects

- Commonly mild, purpuric urticarial papular rash, fever, arthralgia, lymphadenopathy, paresthesia, GI tolerance.
- *Rare but serious side effect*: agranulocytosis, hypothyroidism can occur.

Uses

- Graves' disease.
- Toxic nodular Goiter.
- Preoperatively before surgery.
- Along with ^{131}I.
- *During pregnancy*: Propylthiouracil has maximum protein binding, less chance of placental transfer—hence preferred.

Iodides

- Fastest acting thyroid inhibitor.
- *Mechanism of action*: Iodine is reduced to iodide in the intestine acts by inhibiting release of preformed thyroid hormones.
- Lugol's iodine leads to 5% I_2 + 10% KI is generally used.

Uses

- Preoperative preparation for thyroidectomy given 10 days before operation. It makes gland firm, less vascular, easier to handle.
  - Along with antithyroid drugs in thyroid strom
  - Prophylaxis of endemic goiter
  - As an expectorant
  - Used as antiseptic
  - Used as contrast media
  - To protect thyroid after accidental exposure to radioactive isotopes.

Adverse Effects

- *Acute hypersensitive reaction*: Swelling of lips, eyelids, angioedema, fever, arthralgia, petechial hemorrhage, thrombocytopenia.
- *Chronic uses*: Iodism–metallic taste, inflammation of mucosa, rhinorrhea, sore throat, lacrimation, sneezing, salivation, pulmonary edema.
- *Long-term use*: Hypothyroidism, goiter.
- Flaring of acne.
- In pregnant/nursing mother fetal/infantile goiter.

Preoperative and Perioperative Considerations for Patient with Thyroid Disorder

- Patient should be euthyroid before surgery.
- The elderly hypothyroid patient should be treated with minimum dose of levothyroxine 25 µg/day while 50 µg/day for the adult, gradually increased at 3-4 weekly intervals till euthyroid.
- In case of severe emergency, the hypothyroid patient may be treated with liothyronine (T3) 10-50 µg slow IV under ECG monitoring.
- For the hyperthyroid patient, treatment with carbimazole 30-45 mg orally/day for 6-8 weeks often enables the patient to be euthyroid. Propranolol therapy often becomes necessary for treatment of tremor and palpitations.
- β blockade should continue perioperatively for the hyperthyroid patient to avoid thyroid storm.
- Drug metabolism is slow in the hypothyroid patient, so dose of drugs need to be reduced, titrated accordingly.

CHAPTER 19

Oxygen Therapy and Humidification

INTRODUCTION

The fundamental goal of oxygen therapy is to improve arterial O_2 content. The basic advantages of oxygen therapy are:
- Alveolar O_2 tension is increased.
- Ventilatory work required to maintain a given alveolar O_2 tension is decreased.
- Myocardial work necessary to maintain a given arterial O_2 tension is decreased.

INDICATIONS

- Cardiopulmonary/respiratory arrest.
- Hypoventilation, shock, hemorhage.
- *Cyanosis*: Intracardiac/intrapulmonary shunt.
- LVF, cardiac dysrhythmias.
- COPD, ARDS, atelectasis and severe pneumonia.
- Severe anemia, CO poisoning and cyanide poisoning.
- To decompress distended bowel, surgical emphysema, pneumothorax, air embolism.
- Shivering, hyperthermia and thyroid crisis.

TECHNIQUES OF OXYGEN THERAPY

- **Fixed performance system:**
  - *High flow (HAFOE)*: Ventimask/other venture operated devices allows precise administration of oxygen, tight fitting face mask not required, useful in COPD. Disadvantage is patient cannot eat, drink, talk or cough.
  - *Low flow*: Anesthetic circuit.
- **Variable performance system:**
  - *No capacity system*: O_2 catheter, nasal cannula; advantage-simple to use, high patient acceptibility and comfortable, patients can eat or

drink, flow is 1–6 L/min. Disadvantage—exact concentration of inspired oxygen cannot be achieved.
- *Small capacity system*: Catheter/cannula with high oxygen flow; MC Harris and Edinburg mask. This mask covers nose and mouth, flow is 5–8 L/min, there is chance of rebreathing, removal of mask for a short while will cause sudden steep decrease in PaO_2.
- *Large capacity system*: Pneumask, polymask, BLB, incubator, oxygen tent. These oxygen mask with reservoir deliver > 60% O_2 by a low flow system, flow 6–10 L/min, close fitting mask is provided and one can deliver consistent oxygen concentrate.

- **Special oxygen delivery systems**:
  - O_2 *head hood*: It is used for infants. Oxygen flow is 3 times the minimum volume.
  - *Oxygen tent*: Large capacity system where patient is enclosed. Used in children; air changes of 20 L/hour done.
  - *Oxygen incubator*: Oxygen therapy in a controlled environment of temperature and humidity.
  - *Long-term oxygen therapy*: It is used in patients with chronic hypoxemia like COPD patients; PaO_2 maintained at 60 mm Hg.
  - *C-PAP, BIPAP*: Applied via mask, IPPV—Applied via ventilator.
  - *Transtracheal oxygen delivery*: Via cricothyrotomy membrane puncture. Delivery of O_2 via ETT/tracheostomy tube.
  - *Hyperbaric O_2*: 2–3 ATA pressure O_2 dissolved in plasma increased to 5.5 mL/dL.
  - *ECMO*: Extracorporeal membrane oxygenation.
  - *IVOX*: Intravascular oxygenation.

Clinical Guidance for Oxygen Therapy

Adult with TV = 300–700 mL. Respiration rate <25/min. Ventilation pattern regular-low flow system.

If any one of the above criteria are not fulfilled, high flow system is given.

Evaluation of Effectiveness of Oxygen therapy

- *General*: Pulse, BP, perfusion state and tidal volume, ventilatory rate and work of breathing.
- *Pulse oximetry*: State of oxygenation.
- Arterial blood gas analysis → PaO_2, $PaCO_2$ and pH.

Hazards of Oxygen Therapy

- Abolition of chronic hypoxic respiratory drive in COPD patients → hypercapnea.
- Circulatory depression to abolition of hypoxia-mediated sympathetic activity in some patients.
- Drying and crusting of secretions in respiratory tract—hence the necessity of humidified oxygen.

- *Pulmonary absorption collapse*: Due to high oxygen concentration in lung zones with low ventilation: perfusion v/q areas.
- *Fire and explosion*: Increase in incidence of high concentration of oxygen specially in oxygen tent and pressure chambers.

TOXICITY

Due to free radical injury by superoxide anion, hydrogen peroxide and hydroxyl ion.

- *Pulmonary toxicity*: (Lorrain Smith effect)—due to high concentration of oxygen >48 hours. Resulting in ARDS and pulmonary edema.
- *CNS toxicity (Paul Bert effect)*: High concentration of oxygen >2 ATA pressure will cause; inactivation of GABA resulting in convulsion.
- *Retrolental fibroplasia*: In a healthy person, inspiration of 100% oxygen may be harmful if continued for more than a few hours, 40% can be inhaled indefinitely. The crucial level is determined by arterial PO_2.

HUMIDIFICATION

Normal Mechanics of Humidification

During its passage through the respiratory tract towards the alveoli, inspired gas is brought to body temperature (either by heating/cooling) and 100% relative humidity (either by evaporation or by condensation).

In the unintubated patient, the upper respiratory tract (especially nose) functions as the principal heat and moisture exchanger. Normally, water is lost by the body as saturated vapor in expired gases and heat is lost due to the heat of vaporization for the water supplied by the body. Humidification of O_2 should be considered for patients requiring concentration of O_2 >35%.

Effects of Anesthesia

Water is intentionally removed from the medical gases—(piped/cylinders) to prevent corrosion and condensation in regulators and valves. Thus gases emerging from the anesthesia machine are dry at room temperature. The breathing system, to a considerable extent tracheal tube and the apparatus dead space act as heat and moisture exchanger but of much lower efficacy. Tracheal intubation bypasses the upper respiratory tract—so the burden of humidification and heating falls on the tracheobronchial mucosa.

Effects of Inhaling Dry Gases

- Respiratory mucosa dries—temperature drops, secretions thicken, ciliary function decreases.
- Surfactant activity is impaired.
- Mucosa becomes susceptible to injury.
- Dried secretion cause obstruction to airway, leading to atelectasis.
- Decrease in FRC and reduction in compliance.
- Thickened plugs may provide loci for infection.

- Dry gases can cause bronchoconstrictions. Complete cessation of ciliary activity occurs following prolonged exposure to inspired gas with an absolute humidity below 22 mg/L.
- Body temperature is lowered as the inspired air is humidified and warmed to body temperature—evaporative cooling may result in shivering. This increase in oxygen consumption, increase in carbon dioxide—problem specially in pediatric patient.

Sources of Humidity

- *Carbon dioxide absorbent*: Soda lime reaction liberates water, water is contained in granules.
- *Exhaled gases*: Depending upon the system and amount of rebreathing allowed.
- Rinsing the inside of the breathing tubes and reservoir bag with sterile water before use.

Recommendation for Humidification

- 12–35 mg water/L of O_2. International standard on humidifiers considers 30 mg/L, the minimum amount of humidification necessary to prevent inspiration of secretions and mucosal damage. Air → 44 mg/L, soda lime → 29 mg/L - humidity.
    - *Heat and moisture exchanger humidifier*: Provides relative humidity of 60–70%, temperature of 29–34°C. *Components*: Two ports 15 and 22 mm head with hygrophobic properties (Table 19.1).
      Mechanism: Vol-7.8–59 mL (increase in apparent dead space). Resistance 0.1–2 cm H_2O.

Table 19.1: Advantages and disadvantages of humidifiers and nebulizer.

	Advantage	Disadvantage
Heat and moisture exchanger humidifier	Inexpensive, easy to use, light weight. Does not require water. Does not require extensive energy source. No danger of overhydration. Provided with viral/bacterial filters	Has limited humidity, loss of water from respiratory tract (RT) occurs, relevant only for short procedures, increase in tidal volume (TV), lower the efficiency, increase in resistance
Hot water bath humidifier	Provides fully saturated air at body temperature	It is bulky, difficult to mount, difficult to clean and sterilize, costly, needs electricity, water level to be checked regular and bacterial colonies are predominant
Nebulizers	Deliver saturated vapor without heat. It can produce gases with more water content	Costly, require high gas flow/(gas driven), requires electric (ultrasonic), electrical hazards, water deposit in the tubing of patient

- *Problems*: Resistance, maximum for 24 hours, single patient use. Efficiency decreases with high TV used, gas leak under increase pressure.
- *Hot water bath humidifier*: Used in ICU.
  - *Components*: container with water, thermostatically controlled heating element, tubing to deliver gas, water trap before patient end.
  - *Mechanism*: Fully saturated air at 37°C.
  - Problems are electrical appliance thermostatically controlled, to be positioned below patients airway.
- *Nebulizers*: Produce micro droplets of water of 1-20 diameter. Three types—gas driven nebulizer (2-4 μm), spinning disk nebulizer, and ultrasonic nebulizer (1-2 μm).
- *Entonox*: 50% oxygen and 50% nitrous oxide; delivered during labor or short painful procedures, e.g. fracture reduction; via demand value connected to either face mask or mouth piece.
- *Heliox*: 21% O_2 + 79% helium, allowing faster diffusion of oxygen in a laminar flow, reducing turbulence; used in asthma, COPD, upper airway obstruction etc. Moreover nebulized drugs can be added to Heliox, using helium as a carrier gas.

ANTIOXIDANTS

Antioxidants are believed to quench free radicals. Free radicals are atoms or molecules with singlet/unpaired electron which makes them highly reactive. Oxidative free radicals are generated by metabolic reactions. They create a chain of reactions like lipid peroxidation, DNA damage, etc. Free radicals have been implicated in a variety of disorders, e.g. atherosclerosis, cancers, neurodegenerative disorders and inflammatory bowel diseases.

Endogenous and dietary compounds having antioxidant and free radical scavenging properties are called antioxidants; for example; superoxide dismutase, ferritin, transferrin, ceruloplasmin, α tocopherol, β carotene, Ascorbic acid, glutathione, melatonin and NO.

Based on this theoretical basis, vitamin E, vitamin C, β carotene have been claimed to protect against—atherosclerosis, coronary A disease, CA of breast, lung, mouth, skin, esophagus and stomach.

CHAPTER 20

Drug Therapy in Special Cases

THE PEDIATRIC PATIENTS

PHYSIOLOGY IN THE NEONATE AND PEDIATRIC PATIENTS

Respiratory System (Table 20.1)

At birth, alveoli are thick walled 10% of adult total; lung growth continues till 6-8 years. Airways are relatively narrow, high airway resistance (during anesthesia, resistance to be minimal). Ventilation almost entirely diaphragmatic with ribs being soft and horizontal. High airway resistance and low compliance so ventilatory rate is rapid.

Alveolar minute ventilation is greater but FRC is a similar fraction of lung volume as in adult (so inhalation anesthesia—induction and awakening both are quick).

Physiological dead space 30% of tidal volume as in adult (so during anesthesia dead space should be kept to a minimum). Total and lung dynamic compliance as well as airway conductance related to lung volume (FRC) as in adult but high thoracic compliance. TLC, VC, FRC less per unit body mass in a neonate compared to a child more than 7 years.

Cardiovascular System

The cardiopulmonary circuit flow pattern undergoes a dramatic change after birth; associated with increase in pulmonary blood flow, closure of

Table 20.1: Comparative study of respiratory components in neonate and adult.

	Neonate	Adult
Compliance	5 mL cm H_2O	100 mL cm H_2O
Resistance	30 cm H_2O/sec	2 cm H_2O/L/sec
Time constant	0.5 sec	1.3 sec
Respiratory rate	32/min	15/min

ductus arteriosus and foramen ovale. Decrease in high pulmonary vascular resistance in fetus (Adaptation from fetal to adult type takes first 6 postnatal months).

Myocardial myofilament content increases, maturation of cross bridge attachment, strengthening of cytoskeleton and extracellular (EC) matrix occurs.

Left ventricular wall thickness increases with ECG maturation with left ventricular predominance occurs during 1st year.

Neonate adjusts cardiac output to meet increased metabolic demand by increased heart rate rather than stroke volume (Heart rate less than 20-30% of normal, i.e. less than 100/minute is associated with decrease in CO) can tolerate heart rate till 200/minute. Increase in blood flow to heart, brain and liver compared to other regions. High cardiac output of approx 200 mL/kg/minute which is 2-3 times of an adult. Arrhythmias are uncommon, cardiac arrest usually occurs in asystole.

Systemic arterial pressure is low at birth (80/50 mm Hg) because of low systemic vascular resistance reaches adult value at approximately 16 years of age.

Average blood volume at birth is 90 mL/kg and it decreases to 80 mL/kg in infancy and reaches adult level of 75 mL/kg at 6-8 years. Blood volume loss → 10% should be replaced. Most children with normal Hb can tolerate blood loss of 20%.

A hematocrit of 25% is acceptable. At birth 75-80% of Hb is HbF. HbF has a greater affinity for O_2 due to lower content of 2, 3 DPG and dissociation curve is shifted to left. This is overcome by low PO_2 in tissues and metabolic acidosis helps in O_2 delivery by shifting O_2 dissociation curve to right. (So, hyperventilation → respiratory alkalosis should be avoided during anesthesia as it decreases O_2 availability).

Renal Function and Fluid Balance

Body fluid constitutes a greater proportion of body weight in the infant; ECF/ICF ratio reverse with increase in age. Plasma volume remains constant (5% of body weight) throughout life. Turnover of fluid is more in infants; so water deprivation leads to quick dehydration (15% of total body water/day). At 36 weeks all nephrons are formed but cortical development continues for months (12-24 months). So, kidneys are immature at birth. GFR and tubular reabsorption decreases till 6-8 months, inability to handle excessive water and Na loads. Immature renal function may lead to cumulation and drug toxicity of those drugs excreted by kidneys. Serum levels of electrolytes and osmolality differ little with age but levels of energy ubstrates (glucose, protein) and metabolic products (urea, NPN) increases with age. Large surface area compared to body mass increases evaporative surface area. A healthy infant successfully adjusts its fluid balance and extracellular electrolytes if its birth weight is more than 1500 g. IV fluids should be administered using a burette type of infusion set which should deliver 60 drops/mL.

Temperature Regulation

Neonate has surface area:volume ratio 2.5 times greater than the adult. Heat is lost by conduction, convection and evaporation from skin and respiration tract. Infants less than 3 months old do not shiver and depend on nonshivering (to maintain core temperature of 37°C) thermogenesis—this is achieved by increased metabolism of brown fat (present in neck, upper thoracic area and surrounding great vessels). This metabolism is controlled by sympathetic nervous system; shivering developed by 6 months. Hypothermia may lead to respiratory depression, decrease in cardiac output, prolongation of drug action, increased risk of hypoventilation, regurgitation and aspiration in postoperative (PO) period. O_2 consumption on day 1 of neonate is 5 mL/kg/minute-increases to 7-8 mL/kg/minute by day 7—gradually decreases to adult level of 3-4 mL/kg/minute. Respiratory quotient (VCO_2/VO_2) varies from 0.7 to 1.0 in the neonate. Glucose is the primary energy in the neonate for brain and myocardium. Thermal stress also increases plasma catecholamine causing pulmonary and vascular vasoconstriction and metabolic acidemia.

Heat loss should be prevented in OT by wrapping the limbs in orthopedic wool or padding by using space blanket or silver swaddler, or radiant heaters. Malignant hyperpyrexia is extremely rare less than 3 years of age. Temperature should be monitored; gradients of more than 10°C should be avoided; O_2 consumption increases as temperature difference exceeds 4°C.

Central and Autonomic Nervous System

Neonatal brain receives approx 1/3rd of cardiac output (adult → 1/7 of CO). Autoregulation of global cerebral blood flow. Neurons are developed but myelination is incomplete; BBB is immature so more permeable to drugs including opioids. Majority of body fat in CNS; lipid soluble drugs get easy accessibility—reach high levels easily. Immature CNS → response for increase in MAC of inhalational anesthetics. Parasympathetic system is predominant so bradycardiac response to hypoxemia and other autonomic stimuli, e.g. laryngoscopy. Respond to metabolic stress by increase in plasma levels of catecholamines, adrenocorticosteroids, glucose, insulin and gluconeogenic substrates. Perception of pain developed by the time of viability (24-25 weeks of gestation).

Liver

Qualitative and quantitative difference in plasma protein which decreases in plasma albumin, less protein binding of some drugs, e.g. diazepam and vitamin K can displace bilirubin and cause kernicterus. Enzymes responsible for glucuronidation are immature. Immaturity of liver microsomal enzymes—may be responsible for rarity of halothane induced hepatitis in patients less than 10 years. By 1-2 years liver is twice the volume relative to body weight as in adult.

PHARMACOLOGY OF ANESTHETIC DRUGS

Calculation of pediatric dose:
- Pediatric dose = (Age/Age + 12) × adult dose.
- OR (Age/20) × adult dose.
- **Points to be noted in this respect:**
  - Immature liver, kidney, neuromuscular (NM) junction and enzyme system.
  - Low GFR.
  - Blood–brain barrier is poorly developed.
  - Increased BMR than adults.
  - Tissue blood flow in children is relatively high—quick absorption.

Inhalation Agents

- MAC of anesthetic drugs is higher in infants, e.g. MAC of halothane is 1.1, in adults 0.75.
- Smaller the child, more rapid the uptake.
- High concentration of potent inhalation agents may cause hypotension specially under controlled ventilation.
- Halothane-hepatitis not seen in children less than 14 years.
- Methoxyflurane-induced renal dysfunction is unlikely in children unless a very high dose is needed.

Intravenous Agents

- Preferable for all children more than 3 years.
- Sharp fine-gauge needle no. 26/27.
- Cental venous (CVP) line should never be used.
- Neonates are specially sensitive to barbiturates, of IV agents thiopentone is most popular.
- Methohexital, diazepam, ketamine and althesin has been used.
- Althesin may cause cardiovascular collapse—so has been abandoned.
- Ketamine can be used for superficial operation, specially burn dressing in children, it has no effect on visceral pain, so cannot be used for abdominal surgery.

Precautions Regarding Use of Certain Drugs

- Chloramphenicol can cause 'gray baby syndrome' in premature infants and neonates.
- Sulfonamides may cause kernicterus or severe jaundice.
- Drugs like penicillin, aminoglycosides, sulfonamides, halothane to be used cautiously in premature infants.
- Some drugs like phenytoin, carbamazepine, digoxin may require higher doses.

PATIENT WITH CHRONIC RENAL FAILURE

Chronic renal failure occurs when functioning nephrons are 10-40%. Altered physiological changes associated with more than 90% loss → uremia.

FEATURES ASSOCIATED WITH CHRONIC RENAL FAILURE

- *Anemia*: Hb 5-8 g%. Due to decrease in erythropoietin secretion treated by recombinant human erythropoietin.
  Side effect of erythropoietin—hypertension.
- *Pruritus*: Due to histamine release, relieved by erythropoietin administration.
- *Coagulopathies*: Bleeding tendency due to defective release of von Wilebrand's factor treatment by cryoprecipitate or desmopressin or estrogen therapy. Erythropoietin therapy for anemia shortens bleeding time (BT).
- *Hyperkalemia*: Most serious electrolyte imbalance. Plasma K level of less than 5.5 mg/L is required before administering anesthesia. Treated by—hyperventilation, IV glucose and insulin; IV calcium.
- *Hypocalcemia*: Leading to renal osteodystropy due to hyperphosphatemia, deficiency of vitamin D (active form).
- *Hypermagnesemia*: Due to Mg containing antacids—may lead to depression of CNS.
- *Aluminum-toxicity*: From dialysate fluid or aluminum containing antacids.
- *Metabolic acidosis*: As H^+ ion cannot be properly secreted (normally 50-100 mEq of H^+ ions are secreted).
- *Hypertension*: Due to parenchymal/renovascular cause; activation of renin-angiotensin mechanism is responsible.
- *CVS changes*: CCF, arrhythmias, increase in pericarditis—tamponade and cardiomyopathy.
- *Respiratory changes*: Uremia lung (due to toxic injury), pulmonary edema, pleural effusion and infection.
- *GI system*: Delayed gastric emptying, GI bleeding, nausea, vomiting and diarrhea.
- *Endocrinal changes*: Increase in insulin, increase in glucagon, increase in aldosterone, increase in parathormone, increase in renin, hypothyroidism and hypogonadism.
- *CNS*: CNS depression, encephalopathy, peripheral neuropathies and autonomic (sympathetic) dysfunction.
- *Metabolic*: Hyperlipidemia, glucose intolerance (insulin resistance) and hypoalbuminemia.

PREOPERATIVE PREPARATION

Keeping the above in mind, following prerequisites should be maintained before inducing anesthesia.
- *Hematocrit*: Preferable 30-33%, GA can be administered at 25%. Hb-6-8%.

- Uremic bleeding diathesis should be controlled.
- Plasma K should be less than 5.5 mEq/L.
- Hypertension to be controlled by (to be continued till surgery) either β-blocker/ACE inhibitor.
- If uncontrolled and dialysis is necessary, patient to be put on dialysis, acidosis and electrolyte imbalance is corrected.
- Strict asepsis is to be maintained while placing vascular catheters and endobronchial tube.
- Likelihood of aspiration to be kept in mind.
- Diabetes to be controlled by proper therapy.

Investigations

- Blood Hb%, hematocrit, TC and DC.
- Blood coagulation profile.
- Blood urea nitrogen—most important.
- Serum creatinine—prognostic criteria.
- Serum electrolytes.
- Chest X-ray—To exclude infection and edema.
- ECG—To exclude arrhythmia and cardiomyopathy.

Premedication

- Use of narcotic sedative should be slowly graduated.
- Shorter-acting benzodiazepines, e.g. oxazepam can be given.
- Anticholinergics not indicated.
- NPA, oral cimetidine/rantidine to be given 4 hours preoperatively.

Anesthesia (Table 20.2)

General or regional—any may be given. Induction after proper oxygenation by thiopentone or fentanyl or propofol; etomidate, midazolam can also be given followed by succinylcholine if necessary. Muscle relaxant of choice—atracurium, mivacurium, duration of vecuronium action is less predictable. Anesthesia maintained by O_2, N_2O, isoflurane or halothane or desflurane or short-acting opioid.

Sevoflurane, enflurane are avoided. Intraoperative hypertension can be controlled by vasodilators {cyanide toxicity with sodium nitroprusside (SNP) use is not seen in chronic renal failure (CRF).

Table 20.2: Dose reduction necessary according to rate of creatinine clearance.

Creatinine clearance	Percentage of dose reduction
5–10 mL/min	20%
10–30 mL/min	30%
30–50 mL/min	50%
50–70 mL/min	70%

Normocapnea to be maintained, PEEP should be such that cardiac output is maintained. Intraoperative fluid balance is essential, reversed by glycopyrrolate and neostigmine.

Protocol

- Premedication—midazolam and temazepam.
- Induction—propofol.
- Muscle relaxants—succinylcholine, atracurium and cisatracurium.
- Inhalation agents—isoflurane, desflurane and halothane.
- Local anesthetics—25% reduced dose of bupivacaine and lidocaine.
- Analgesic—paracetamol.
- Monitoring—pulse, BP, PAWP, CVP (10 cm during revascularization), pulseoximtery, H_2O, ECG, temperature, urine output (more than 0.5 mL/kg/hr).

POSTOPERATIVE FOLLOW-UP

- Hypertension to be controlled.
- Fluid balance to be maintained.
- Urine output to be noted.
- Postoperative assessment of serum K, glucose, Hb% as well as electrolytes.

Precautions to be Taken for Drug Therapy of Following Drugs

- Drugs causing direct injury, e.g. NSAIDs, aminoglycosides and heavy metals.
- Dose adjustment necessary for drugs like atenolol, acebutolol, warfarin, diazepam, digoxin and phenobarbitone.
- Thiazides to be avoided in renal failure and may cause exacerbation.
- Uricosuric drugs are ineffective, so should be avoided.
- Nephrotoxic drugs like tetracyclines, sulfonamides, aminoglycosides, cephalexin, vancomycin, amphotericin B, ethambutol, acyclovir should better be avoided.
- CNS depressants like benzodiazepines, barbiturates, pethidine may produce enhanced CNS depression.
- Antihypertensives may produce more postural hypotension.

DOSE CALCULATION IN IMPAIRED RENAL FUNCTION

$$\text{Dose in renal impaired patient} = \frac{\text{Creatinine clearance in renal impaired}}{\text{Creatinine clearance in normal subject}}$$

- Creatinine clearance can be calculated by Cockroft Gault formula;
  - Creatinine clearance(mL/min) =
  $$\frac{(140 - \text{age}) \times \text{weight (kg)} \times (0.85 \text{ for women})}{72 \times \text{serum creatinine (mg/dL)}}$$

PATIENT WITH LIVER DYSFUNCTION

PATHOPHYSIOLOGICAL CHANGES ASSOCIATED WITH CHRONIC LIVER DISEASE

- *Ascites*: Due to Na and H_2O retention as a result of activation of renin-angiotensin system. Ascites may cause respiratory embarrassment by diaphragmatic splinting, decrease in functional residual capacity (FRC), decrease in tidal volume (TV). Treatment with Na restriction, potassium sparing diuretic; paracentesis in refractory cases should be done 12 hours before surgery.
- *Pulmonary system*: Increase in intrapulmonary shunt, pulmonary hypertension, increase in CO, pleural effusion, hypoxia and hyperventilation.
- *CVS changes*: Hyperdynamic circulation, increase in cardiac output, increase in systemic vascular resistance (SVR), left ventricular dysfunction, alcoholic cardiomyopathy.
- *Kidney*: Dilutional hyponatrema and hepatorenal syndrome.
- *Coagulation*: Increase in PT, platelet count decrease. Treatment done with vitamin K 10 mg TDS IM × 3 days preoperatively. FFP increase in coagulation factors except F XIII (which is replaced by cryoprecipitate).
- *Cause of death*: Hemorrhage, sepsis, renal failure and encephalopathy.
- *Metabolic*: Metabolic alkalosis, hyperglycemia and encephalopathy.
  In severe cases: Metabolic acidosis.
- *Altered drug response*: Resistance to sedatives, oxidative enzymes decrease resulting in prolonged drug effect, resistance to neuromuscular agents. ECF increase due to greater volume of distribution–serum albumin decrease, increase in free drug. Renal impairment will impair elimination, with increase in chance of drug toxicity.

PREOPERATIVE PREPARATION

- *Assess patient*: Grade according to Child's criteria.
- Preoperative vitamin K.
- Preoperative paracentesis, if required.
- Hydrate patient.
- *Premedicants avoided*: Opioids avoided.
- Gut sterilization, midazolam.
- Serum electrolytes, pH, blood and gas analysis.
- Anemia treated.

Anesthesia (Drugs Recommended)

- *Premedication*: Lorazepam.
- *Inducing agent*: Propofol, thiopentone.
- *Neuromuscular agent*: Atracurium or vecuronium.
- *Opioids if required*: Remifentanil.
- *Inhalation if required*: Isoflurane, desflurane, sevoflurane.
- *Analgesic*: Paracetamol.

POSTOPERATIVE FOLLOW-UP
- Urine output.
- Antibiotic cover.

Precautions to be Taken Regarding Drug Therapy
- Dose of drugs like lignocaine, morphine, propranolol and drugs which are entirely metabolized in the liver, should be reduced.
- Drugs with short half-life and minimum hepatic metabolism to be preferred, e.g. oxazepam/lorazepam in place of diazepam.
- Drugs which cause direct hepatic injury, e.g. paracetamol, salicylates, tetracyclines, steroids, halothane, methyldopa, INH, dantrolene to be avoided.
- Liver damage may cause increased plasma concentration of drugs either due to diminished first pass metabolism or decreased plasma-protein binding.
- Prodrugs, necessitating hepatic metabolism and activation needs to be avoided.
- Plasma concentration of electrolytes to be measured if diuretic therapy becomes necessary, potassium sparing diuretics are preferred as hypokalemic alkalosis leads to conversion of NH_4^+ to NH_3 which easily crosses BBB resulting in mental alteration.
- Oral anticoagulants to be used cautiously as coagulation factors are low.
- Enhanced fluid retention due to NSAIDs and increased incidence of lactacidosis due to metformin.
- The dictum of drug therapy is minimum drugs at minimum dose and which are essentially necessary should only be prescribed.

THE ELDERLY PATIENT

Old age is associated with increase in heterogenicity in responses to medications presumptively related to—
- Age related comorbidities.
- Use of multiple medications.
- Interindividual variability in the effects of aging on pharmacokinetic and pharmacodynamic processes.

AGE-RELATED CHANGES IN PHARMACOKINETICS AND PHARMACODYNAMICS

The doses of many drugs should be reduced in older people to compensate for the age-related changes in pharmacokinetics specially renal function.
- Glomerular filtration rate (GFR) decreases slowly from about 20 years of age, falling by about 25% at 50 years and 50% by 75 years. This closely correlates with creatinine clearance. Plasma creatinine typically remains with in the normal adult range despite decrease in GFR; this can be explained by their decrease in muscle mass.
- Changes in drug absorption from the gut, protein binding and volume of distribution.
- Hepatic metabolism of drugs is reduced. The activity of hepatic microsomal enzymes declines slowly with age.
- Distribution of volume of lipid-soluble drugs is increased, because the proportion of the body fat increases with advancing age, e.g. increase in plasma half-life of diazepam with advancing age.
- There is variability in plasma half-life of drugs between individuals with increasing age.
- Age-related variation in sensitivity of drugs, e.g. diazepam causes more confusion in elderly compared to the young; hypotensive drugs cause postural hypotension more in elderly.
- The prevalence of adverse drug reactions is increased in the elderly. About 80% of adverse drug reactions in elderly are of type A.
- At least 5 steps should be undertaken by clinicians while prescribing for the elderly:
  - Determination of the efficacy of the medicine
  - Determination of the likely adverse effects
  - Discussions of risk benefit with the patient
  - Decision of the dose regime
  - Monitoring of the patient during the therapy.

The prevalence of adverse effects is increased in the elderly and reactions are generally more severe. Aging process is not an independent risk factor, but merely a marker for comorbidity, altered pharmacokinetics and polypharmacy has been considered most important. As the type of adverse reactions is of type A, it should be taken to be predictable and preventable by:
- Meticulous approach to risk benefit ratio prior to embarking pharmacotherapy.

- Dosage adjustment should be based on the altered patterns of drug disposition and pharmacodynamic response in the elderly. Adverse effects are more common with certain drugs, e.g. NSAID specially COX-2 selective agents → upper GI hemorrhage, perforation and hypertension.
    - H_2 receptor antagonists → idiosyncriatic reactions including intestinal nephritis, hepatitis.
    - Bisphosphonates → adverse GI symptoms, e.g. esophageal ulceration and stricture. Risedronate seems to have less GI symptoms compared to alendronate.
    - Benzodiazepines. Incidence of sedation and confusion → falls.
    - SSRI.
    - Newer antipsychotics
        - However increase in incidence of falls is not seen with diuretics, β-blockers, centrally acting antihypertensives, ACE inhibitors, calcium channel blockers and nitrates.
        - Polypharmacy exacerbates risk of delirium. Polypharmacy is defined as use of >5 medications. Anticholinergic drugs and psychotropic drugs are frequently recognized as causing confusion.

Principles to be followed to prevent complications are—
- Polypharmacy should be avoided—it should be only done when indication is therapeutically compelling, clinician can monitor and access comparative benefit and safety of the patient. There is well established clinical trial evidence base.
- Therapeutic drug monitoring to be applied where indicated.
- Dose monitoring —dictum to be followed is 'start low, go slow.'

DRUGS WITH REDUCED RENAL OR HEPATIC ELIMINATION IN THE ELDERLY

- Antibiotics like penicillin, tetracyclines and aminoglycosides.
- Sedative hypnotics like diazepam, alprazolam, barbiturates and nitrazepam.
- Antihypertensives like propranolol, atenolol, clonidine, lisinopril, captopril, enalapril and guanfacine.
- NSAIDs, diuretics, theophylline, warfarin and digoxin.
- Cimetidine, ranitidine and famotidine.
- Lithium and antidepressants.

CHAPTER 21

Management of Emergency Situations

ACUTE SEVERE ASTHMA

Monitoring of peak flow rate is essential for diagnosis. A peak flow rate of less than 30% of normal, PaO_2 less than 60 mm Hg and a rising $PaCO_2$ are typical.

Management

- High flow and moist O_2 inhalation.
- Nebulized β_2-agonists like salbutamol or terbutaline 5 mg in 3 mL of normal saline, repeated every 1–2 hours till symptoms are controlled.
- IV hydrocortisone 200 mg 8 hourly.
- Aminophylline 6 mg/kg body weight in 20 mL of 5% dextrose IV slowly over 20 minutes.
- Nebulized ipratropium bromide 500 µg 6 hourly.
- In acute cases, adrenaline 0.5 mL of 1:1000 solution SC to a maximum of 2 mL.
- Ventilatory support, if necessary.

HYPERTENSIVE CRISIS

This situation can arise in patients who have preexisting hypertension and occasionally in normotensive patients, when BP may shoot up to 250 mm Hg systolic or 120–130 mm Hg diastolic. Such rise can also occur on sudden withdrawal of antihypertensive like clonidine or β-blockers. Management depends on quick assessment and immediate treatment. The drugs, listed in the further given table, can be used.

Drug	Dose	Onset of action	Duration of action
Sodium nitroprusside	0.25–10 µg/kg/min IV infusion given via microdrip	Immediate	1–3 min
Nitroglycerin	5–100 µg/kg/min IV infusion	2–5 min	1–3 min
Diazoxide	15–30 mg/min IV infusion or 50 mg IV bolus dose, repeated at 5–10 minute intervals	1–2 min	6–8 hrs
Esmolol	500 µg/kg/min for 4 min, followed by 150–300 µg/kg/min IV infusion	1–2 min	8–10 min
Labetalol	2 mg/min IV infusion or 20–80 mg IV bolus dose, repeated every 10 min	5–10 min	3–6 hrs
Hydralazine	10–20 mg IV or 10–50 mg IM	10–20 min	3–6 hrs
Nicardipine	5–15 mg/hr followed by 3–8 mg/hr IV.	1–3 min	15–40 min
Enalaprilat	0.625–1.25 mg IV bolus 6 hourly	10–15 min	6–8 hrs
Phentolamine	5–15 mg IV	1–2 min	10–30 min
Trimethaphan	1–4 mg/min IV infusion	1–5 min	5–10 min
Propranolol	1–5 mg IV bolus followed by 3 mg/hr	1–2 min	3–6 hrs

Acute Myocardial Infarction

- Supportive therapy—
  - Complete bedrest; moist oxygen.
  - *Morphine*: 2 mg IV or buprenorphine 0.3 mg.
  - 5% dextrose drip.
  - Isosorbide dinitrate 10 mg 8 hourly.
  - IV nitroglycerin 5-10 µg/min.
  - β-blockers if not C/I can be given within first 6 hours of infarction; metoprolol 1-5 mg or esmolol 50-200 µg/kg/min.
- Interventional therapy—
  - Alteplase 15 mg IV bolus, followed by 50 mg over 30 minutes, given preferably within 6 hours of infarction.
  - Heparin 5000 units in bolus IV followed by 1000 units/hour (PTT to be kept at 1.5-2 times control level. LMW heparins may also be used).
  - Aspirin 165-325 mg orally or clopidogrel 75-600 mg.

SEVERE LARYNGOSPASM

Barbiturate anesthesia, lighter planes of anesthesia, intense surgical stimuli, accumulation of tracheobronchial secretions or hypocalcemia may induce acute laryngospasm often noticed during reversal phase of anesthesia.

Management
- Removal of precipitating factor.
- High concentration of oxygen.

- Suxamethonium 0.25-0.5 mg/kg IV relieves the spasm; or else 2-4 mg/kg IM.
- Topical lignocaine spray, maximum 4 mg/kg, prior to intubation, if necessary.

PULMONARY EDEMA

May follow acute left ventricular failure, aspiration, acute laryngospasm with airway obstruction, fluid overloading.

Management

- High flow 100% O_2 inhalation.
- Optimization of fluid therapy.
- Furosemide 50 mg IV.
- Morphine 5 mg IV.
- GTN infusion under invasive BP monitoring.

MALIGNANT HYPERTHERMIA

Unexplained tachycardia, masseter spasm, generalized muscle rigidity, rising end tidal CO_2, falling PaO_2 with rise of core temperature at the rate of 2°C per hour following administration of suxamethonium or volatile agents like halothane indicates occurrence of malignant hyperthermia.

Management

- Removal of offending agent.
- Airway, breathing, circulation.
- 100% oxygen therapy.
- Dantrolene sodium 2-3 mg/kg IV maximum 10 mg/kg.
- Surgery to be stopped or to be done under total intravenous anesthesia and TIVA.
- Ice-cold fluid IV, intraperitoneally-ice-cold sponging.
- Correction of acidosis or hyperkalemia if necessary.

RAISED INTRACRANIAL PRESSURE

- *Hypernventilation*: Reduction of $PaCO_2$ by 5-10 mm Hg reduces ICP by 25-30%.
- *Mannitol*: 0.25 g/kg IV every 3-5 hours depending on ICP.
- IV dexamethasone 4-6 mg 6 hourly.
- Thiopentone 1-5 mg/kg, may be repeated in small doses.
- Maintenance therapy with fluid restriction and sedation. Muscle relaxation, BP control, prevention of seizures or high fever. Head elevation to 30° may have beneficial effect.

ACUTE ADRENAL CRISIS

- IV hydrocortisone 200 mg stat followed by 100 mg 6 hourly in first 24-48 hours. Then oral prednisolone with a mineralocorticoid.

- Fluid and electrolyte balance; 2L of NS in first 24 hours and 1L of 5% dextrose. Inotropes and vasoconstrictors are often required.
- Correction of hypokalemia, if present.
- Diagnosis and correction of precipitating factors.

THYROID STORM

- *Propylthiouracil*: Loading dose of 600 mg followed by 250 mg 6 hourly.
- Methimazole/Carbimazole may be given 20 mg 3-4 times/day.
- Sodium iodide 1 g in 500 mL dextrose over 8-12 hours; maximum 3 g, maintenance dose of 0.5 g daily for next 2 days.
- Propranolol 1 mg in incremental dose till 10 mg under CVS monitoring. Hydrocortisone 100 mg IV 8 hourly routinely till crisis is controlled.
- Fluid and electrolyte balance; 3-4 L in 24 hours.
- O_2 at the rate of 6-8 L/min.
- Correction of hyponatremia, hypokalemia, if present.
- Phenobarbitone 60 mg IM, if patient is restless; repeated, if necessary.
- Symptomatic relief of hyperpyrexia.

CARDIAC ARREST

- Verify the situation; look for breathing and pulse.
- High-quality CPR with minimal interruption.
- Follow AHA algorithm for basic life support; maintenance of B (breathing), A (airway), C (circulation); adequate oxygenation.
- *Vasopressor therapy*: Inj adrenaline 1 mg in dilution, every 3-5 minutes with vasopressin 40 IU, repeated once or twice shock, if necessary. Defibrillation/shock; CPR to continue in between shock. Atropine 1 mg, repeated if necessary in asystole.
- After third shock, amiodarone 300 mg may be required; lidocaine in VT or Mg in torsades de pointes.

Treatment of Drug Overdose

Drug	Antidote
Benzodiazepines	Flumazenil IV 0.1 mg → 0.2 mg → 0.3 mg → 0.5 mg as required
Atropine	Physostigmine 0.02 mg/kg or 0.5 mg IV/IM/SC repeated to a max. of 2 mg as required
Calcium channel blockers	10% calcium gluconate 100 mg/kg IV or 10% Calcium chloride 20 mg/kg
Metoclopramide (EPS)	Diphenhydramine 1-2 mg/kg IV may be repeated at 30 min interval, max. 300 mg/day
Heparin	Protamine sulfate 2.5-5 mg/kg; 1 mg for every 100 units of heparin

Contd...

Contd...

Drug	Antidote
Warfarin	Vitamin K 5–10 mg IM/IV
Opioids	Naloxone hydrochloride 0.1 mg/kg IV repeated at 2–3 min interval to a max. of 2–4 mg
Beta blockers	Atropine 0.02 mg/kg SC to a maximum of 2 mg

Bibliography

1. Allman KG, Wilson IH. Oxford Handbook of Anaesthesia, 3rd edition. New York: Oxford University Press. 2011. pp. 42-285.
2. Davey AJ, Diba A. Ward's Anesthetic Equipment, 6th edition. China: Elsevier Publishing Division. 2012. pp. 207-22.
3. John MS, Harris RA. Hypnotics and sedatives. In: Brunton L, Chabner B, Knollman B (editors). Goodman & Gilman's: The Pharmacological Basis of Therapeutics, 12th edition. New York: McGraw-Hil Medical Publishing Division. 2011. pp. 457-80.
4. Miller RD. Anaesthetic pharmacology. In: Miller's Anaesthesia, 7th edition. USA: Churchill Livingstone-Elsevier. 2010. pp. 479-957.
5. Miller RD, Pardo MC Jr. Basics of Anesthesia, 6th edition. Haryana: Elservier Publishing Division. 2017. pp. 717-28.
6. Singh M, Deorari A. Drug Dosages in Children, 8th edition. New Delhi: Sagar Publications. 2011. pp. 18-130.
7. Stoelting RK, Hillier SC. Pharmacology and Physiology in Anaesthetic Practice, 4th edition. Philadelphia, USA: Lippincott Williams and Wilkins. 2006.
8. Trevor AJ, Way WL. Sedative-hypnotic drugs. In: Katzung BG, Masters SB, Trevor AJ (editors). Basic and Clinical Pharmacology, 12th edition. New Delhi: Tata McGraw Hil Publishing Division. 2012. pp. 373-88.
9. Tripathi KD. Sedative-hypnotics. In: Essentials of Medical Pharmacology, 6th edition. New Delhi: Jaypee Brothers Medical Publishers (P) Ltd. 2008. pp. 388-400.
10. Udwadia FE. Cardiovascular problems requiring critical care and organ system dysfunction requiring critical care. In: Principles of Critical Care, 2nd edition. New Delhi: Oxford University Press. 1999. pp. 171-220 and 535-77 respectively.

Index

Page numbers followed by *f* refer to figure, *fc* refer to flowchart, and *t* refer to table.

A

Abciximab 192
Acetaminophen 72
　side effect 73
　toxicity 73
Acetic acid derivatives 69
Acetylation 18
Acetylcholine 13
　action of 61
　receptors for 9
Acetylcysteine 126
Acid-base
　and electrolyte balance 72
　imbalance 179
Adenosine 185, 186
　monophosphate 120
　　cyclic 10
　triphosphate 13, 18
Adrenal crisis, acute 231
Adrenaline 131, 132, 146, 150
Adrenergic receptors 8
Adrenocorticotropic hormone 78
Adverse drug reaction 19, 22
Aerosol 123
　therapy 119
Agonist
　antagonists 84
　full 8
　partial 8
Alcohol, acute ingestion of 208
Alcoholic beverages 46
Aldosterone 154
　antagonist 162, 163
Alkaloids
　atropine, natural 65*t*
　natural 65
　pilocarpine 1
Allergic reactions, drug-induced 22
Allopurinol 17

Alosetron 104
Alpha glucosidase inhibitors 208
Alprazolam 48, 52, 102, 228
Alteplase 193
Aluminum hydroxide 110, 114
Aluminum-toxicity 222
Alveolar concentration, minimum 25
Alveolar minute ventilation 218
Amantadine 198
American Thoracic Society 115
Amethocaine 91, 93
Amiloride 163
Amineptine 200
Amino acid sequence 16
Aminophylline 117
Aminosteroid 53
Amiodarone 186
Amitriptyline 201
Amlodipine 158, 174
　felodipine 151
Ammonio steroid compounds 54
Amoxapine 201
Amrinone 132, 150
Analgesia 69
　patient-controlled 77
　stage of 27
Analgesics 76
　centrally acting 78
Anaphylactic shock, treatment of 133
Anemia 222
Anesthesia 49, 225
　clinical signs of 27
　effects of 215
　for hypertensive patients,
　　management of 159
　mechanism of 27
　precautions during 184
　stage of surgical 28
Anesthetic agent 40*t*
　ideal 35

Anesthetic drugs, pharmacology of 221
Anesthetic implications 205
Anesthetize mucous membranes 90
Angina
    drugs in 160
    pectoris, worsening of 120
    unstable 160
Angioedema 172
Angiotensin converting enzyme 153, 167
    inhibitors 153, 166, 170
        side effects of 171f
Angiotensin II receptor blockers 172
Angiotensin peptides 167
Angiotensin receptor blockers 151, 153
Angiotensinogen 166
Antacids 114
Antagonists, receptor 103
Antiadrenergic drugs 104, 109, 122, 155, 228
Antiarrhythmic drugs
    classification of 185
    efficacy of 186
Antiarrhythmics 178
Anti-asthma drugs, comparison of 117t
Anticholinergic drugs 67t, 228
    in anesthesia 65
Anticholinesterases 63t
Anticoagulants agent 187
Anticonvulsant 49, 200
Antidepressants
    atypical 200, 202
    long-term effects of 201
    mechanism of action of 200t
    tricyclic 202
Antidiabetic agents 209t
Antidiabetic drugs 206
Antiemetics 205
Antiepileptic drugs 205
Antihistamines 128
Antihistaminics drugs 104
Antihypertensive 154t, 159t
    action 151f
Anti-inflammatory drugs, nonsteroidal 68, 166
Antiplatelet agent 187
Antipsychotics, newer 228
Antipyresis 69
Antithyroid drugs 211

Antitussives 127
Anxiety 143
Apixaban 191
Apomorphine 196
Ardeparin 189
Argatroban 190
Arrhythmias 120
Arterial blood pressure 166
Arterial hypoxemia 180
Arterial pressure, mean 40, 131
Arylacetic acid derivatves 69
Ascites 225
Aspiration pneumonia 111
Aspirin 70, 191
    therapy, high dose 208
Asthma
    acute severe 125, 229
    drugs in treatment of 115
    grades of 116t
Atenolol 144, 156
    acebutolol 151
Atherosclerosis 217
Athletic heart syndrome 180
Atracurium 53, 55
Atrial fibrillation 182
Atrial flutter 182
Atrial premature beat 181
Atrial septal defect 184
Atrioventricular heart block
    second-degree 178
    third-degree 179
Atropine 1, 67, 232
    flush 66
    methonitrate 65
    sulfate 67
Attack, prevention of future 161
Autonomic ganglia 54, 155

B

Bambuterol 117, 120
Barbiturate 36, 46, 47, 49, 51, 228
    anesthesia 230
Bartter syndrome 71
Beclomethasone dipropionate 117
Bendrofluazide 163
Benzocaine 90
Benzodiazepines 46, 47, 52, 107, 228, 232
    newer 52
Benztropine 198

Benzylisoquinolines 53
Beta-blockers 140, 151, 152, 156, 166, 208, 233
  actions of 142f
  generation 141fc
  mechanisms of action of 144
  nonselective 140fc
  selective 140fc
  use of 144
Beta$_2$-selective agonists, types of 119fc
Beta-endorphin 79
Betamethasone 15
Bifascicular heart block 179
Bioavailability 2
  influence 4
Biotransformation 15
  reactions 15
  types 16
Bisoprolol 156
Bisphosphonates 228
Bivalirudin 190
Bladder 146
Blood glucose 207
  level 210
    monitoring 210t
Blood potassium level 210
  monitoring 210t
Blood pressure
  factors influencing 152fc
  management protocol 153
Blood vessels 146
Blood-brain barrier 62, 195
Bradycardia, management of 132
Bradycardia-tachycardia syndrome 181
Bradykinesia 198
Brain 15
  neonatal 220
Brainstem centers 101
Bromhexine 126
Bromide 46
Bronchial asthma
  classification of drugs in 116
  drugs for 115
Bronchodilators 116
  mechanism of action of 118f
Budesonide 117
Bumetanide 163
Bupivacaine 88, 89, 91, 92
Buprenorphine 84
Bupropion 200

Buspirone 51
Butorphanol 84

C

Caffeine 17, 21, 120, 121
Calcium 18
  carbonate 114
  channel blockers 124, 138, 151, 153, 158, 173, 174t, 232
    actions of 173t
  channels, types of 173t, 174
Calmodulin 19
Cancers 217
Candesartan 172
Captopril 134, 157, 170
Carbamazepine 17
Carbidopa 195
Carbocisteine 126
Carbon dioxide 34
  absorbent 216
Carcinogenesis 21
Cardiac arrest 232
Cardiac arrhythmia 60, 143
Cardiac dysrhythmia 178, 179
Cardiac glycosides 176, 176t
  mechanism of action of 176fc
Cardiac insufficiency 129
Cardiac rhythm, disturbances of 180, 180fc
Cardiac surgery 182
Cardic output 40
Cardiovascular structure, alteration of 169
Cardiovascular system 24, 49, 218
  drugs acting in 129
Catecholamine 180
  types of 131fc
Catechol-o-methyltransferase 195, 197
Ceiling diuretics, high 162
Celiprolol 144
Cellular proteins 13
Central and autonomic nervous system 220
Central nervous system 12, 13, 46, 78, 146, 195, 202
  action on 62, 65
  drugs in 195
  toxicity 215
  type 14
Central venous pressure 131

Cerebral blood flow 40
Cerebral metabolic rate 40
Cervical cord injury, high 130
Chemical stability 4
Chlophedianol 128
Chloral hydrate 17, 46
Chloramphenicol 17
Chlordiazepoxide 46, 48
Chloroprocaine 91
Chlorpromazine 5, 198
Chlorthalidone 163
Cholinergic agents 65
Cilnidipine 175
Cimetidine 17
Cinnarizine 105
Cisapride 106
Cis-atracurium 53, 55
Citalopram 200
Clarithromycin 17
Clomipramine 201
Clonazepam 49, 52
Clonidine 45, 151
Clopidogrel 192
Clozapine 17
Coagulopathy 222
Cocaine 89, 92
Codeine 17, 78, 81, 82, 128
Colloidal bismuth 113
Concomitant disease 159
Congeners, uses of 84
Congestive heart failure 137, 138, 153
  treatment of 138
Conn's syndrome 151
Conscious sedation 44
Coronary syndrome, acute 136
Coronary vessels, vasospasm of 160
Corticosteroids 102, 116, 208
Cortisol 15
Cough 126, 172
  center 126
  drugs in 126
  inability to 95
Cromolyn sodium 123
Cushing's syndrome 17
Cyclizine 105
Cyclooxygenase 68, 69
  inhibitors, nonselective 69
Cytochrome 16
Cytokines 68

D

Dabigatran etexilate 191
Dalteparin 189
Desflurane 31
Desirudin 190
Dexamethasone 102, 107
Dexloxiglumide 107
Dexmedetomidine 44, 45
Dextromethorphan 128
Diabetes, insulin in treatment of 206
Diabetic ketoacidosis 207
Diabetic patient
  perioperative steps for 210
  preoperative steps for 210
Diacylglycerol 11, 19
Dialysis disequilibrium syndrome 165
Diaphragm 126
Diazepam 44, 48, 49, 52, 205, 220, 226, 228
Diazoxide 157, 230
Dibucaine 91
Diclofenac 74
  sodium 67
Dicyclomine 105
Dietary salt intake 166
Diflunisal 72
Digitalis 132, 186
  toxicity 177
Digitoxin 176, 176t
Digoxin 114, 150, 176, 176t
  pharmacokinetics of 177
  therapy, disadvantages of 177
Dihydropyridines 174
Diligan 108
Diltiazem 158, 174, 186
Dipeptidyl peptidase 208
Diphenhydramine 232
Dipyridamole 192
Disopyramide 186
Disulfiram 17
Diuretics 151, 153, 154, 162, 162t
  commonly used 163t
  comparison of 162t
  sites of action of 164f
Dobutamine 131, 132, 148, 150
Domperidone 67, 103, 108
Donepezil 61
Dopamine 131, 132, 147, 150, 198
  agonists 198

receptor
  agonists 196
  distribution of 199
Dopexamine 131, 132
Doxacurium 53, 55
Doxazosin 156
Doxepin 201
Doxinate 108
Doxylamine 105, 108
Dronabinol 107
Droperidol 42
Drug 1, 42
  absorption of 2
  action, targets for 13
  active principle of 1
  administration, routes of 1, 2fc
  agonism 8
    types of 8fc
  allergic reaction to 22
  antagonism 6, 6fc, 7f
    chemical 6
    competitive 7, 7f
    functional 7
    irreversible 7
    noncompetitive 7, 7f
    pharmacokinetic 6
    physiological 7
    receptor block 6
    reversible 7
  application, routes of 2f
  causes, sudden withdrawal of 143
  centrally acting 152
  commonly used 110t
  for cough, classification of 126fc
  interaction 86, 208
  methods to ensure safety of 5
  midazolam, bioavailability of 3f
  names of 1
  overdose, treatment of 232
  pH of 4
  properties of 1
  reactions, allergic 20
  risk-free 5
  routes, determination of 1
  safety profile of 4
  solubility of 4
  therapy 160, 218, 224, 226
Drug-drug interactions 20
D-tubocurarine 53
Ductus arteriosus, action on 70

Dynorphin A 79
Dysgeusia 172
Dyskinesia 196
Dyspepsia 114
Dyspnea, drugs for 128

E

Ebstein's anomaly 181, 184
Ecothiophate 61
Edrophonium 61
Effector cell 11
Emergency situations, management of 229
Enalapril 151, 157, 170
Enalaprilat 157, 230
Endocrinal changes 222
Endocrine
  effects 142
  system, drugs acting on 206
Endogenous opioid system 78
Enflurane 31, 205
Enoxaparin 189
Entonox 217
Enzymes 15
Ephedrine 120
Epidermal growth factor 8
Epidural anesthesia, complications of 95t
Epidural block 99
Epidural injection, therapeutic of 100
Epilepsy 205
Epinephrine 120
Eplerenone 163
Epoxide hydrolases 16
Erythromycin 17
Escitalopram 200
Eserine 61
Esmolol 144, 230
Esophageal ulceration 228
Eszopiclone 52
Ethacrynic acid 163
Ethanol 17
Ether anesthesia, based on 27
Etidocaine 92
Etomidate 38, 40, 205
Etorphine 79
Excitement, stage of 28
Exhaled gases 216

Extradural anesthesia, contraindications for 96
Extrapyramidal syndrome 199
Eye 22, 142
    action on 62, 66

F

Famotidine 67, 110
Fat-soluble vitamins 114
Felodipine 174
Fenamates 69
Fentanyl 41, 42, 44, 67, 79, 83
Fibrinolytics agent 193, 187
Fire and explosion 215
Flecainide 186
Fluid
    balance 219
    therapy 130
Flumazenil 232
Fluoroquinolones 114
Fluoxetine 200
Flurazepam 48, 52
Flurbiprofen 75
Fluticasone propionate 117
Fluvoxamine 200
Fondaparinux 189
Formoterol 120
Fosinopril 170
Fracture reduction 217
Furosemide 163, 208

G

Ganglia, action on 62
Gantacurium 55
Gas effect, second 32
Gastric acid 66
    secretion 109
        reduction of 109
Gastric irritant 127
Gastrointestinal tract 5, 15, 106
    action in 66, 70
General anesthetics 24
    components of 25
    history 24
    physiological effects of 24
General pharmacology 1
Genetic polymorphism 17
Genleuton 123
Glaucoma 143
Glibenclaminde 209
Gliclazide 209
Glimeperide 209
Glipizide 209
Glomerular filtration rate 227
Glucocorticoids 17, 122
Glucose 219
    absorption, decreases 209
Glucuronic acid 18
Glutathione conjugation 15
Glycemic goals, preoperative 206
Glyceryl trinitrate 134-136
Glycine conjugation 18
Glycopyrrolate 67, 184
Glycoside 176
Glycosuria 209
G-protein 9
    coupled receptor 8, 9, 11
    activation of 9
Granisetron 67, 104, 108
Gravidox 108
Griseofulvin 17
Growth hormone 8
Guanethidine 151
Guanosine
    diphosphate 10
    triphosphate 9, 10

H

H_2 antagonists 110
Halothane 29, 226
    actions 29
    hepatitis syndrome 30
Head injury, severe 130
Headache 95
Heart 12, 146
    block
        complete 132
        unifascicular 178
    failure
        beta blockers in 144
        vasodilators in 137
    rate 40
Heliox 217
Helium 34
Hematological reactions, drug-induced 22
Heparin 187, 189, 232
    antagonist 191
    treatment 187

Hepatic disease 5
Hepatic metabolism 227
Hiccups 95
His-Purkinje conduction system 178
Histamine release 54
Hot water bath humidifier 217
Human insulins 206
Human liver, metabolism in 16
Humidification 215, 216
    normal mechanics of 215
Humidifiers and nebulizer
    advantages of 216*t*
    disadvantages of 216*t*
Humidity, sources of 216
Hydralazine 134, 136, 151, 157, 230
Hydrochlorothiazide 151, 163
Hydrogen sulfide 34
Hydromorphone 79
Hyoscine 65*t*, 67, 105, 108
    butylbromide 65
Hypercarbia 180
Hyperkalemia 60, 222
Hypermagnesemia 222
Hyperosmolar nonketotic coma 207
Hypersensitive reaction, acute 212
Hypertension 151, 180, 222
    classification of 153*t*
    drugs in 151, 152
Hypertensive crisis 229
Hyperthermia 180
    malignant 231
Hypnotics 46
    newer 50
Hypocalcemia 222
Hypoglycemia 208
Hypokalemia, acute 180
Hypotension 95
Hypothermia 25
Hypovolemia 129
Hypoxia, diffusion 33

I

Iatrogenic disease 5
Ibuprofen 17, 74
    side effect 74
Idraparinux 189
Imipramine 201
Inadequate anesthesia 95
Indapamide 151, 163

Indomethacin 73, 114
Inflammatory bowel diseases 217
Inhalation
    agents 221
    anesthesia 218
    side effect of 119
Inhalational anesthesia, principles of 27
Inhalational steroids 123
    side effects of 123
Inhalers used, types of 119
Inhaling dry gases, effects of 215
Inositol triphosphate 11
Inotropic agents and vasoconstrictors 146
Insulin 8, 15
    allergy 208
    analogs 206
    aspart 206
    delivery devices 207
    glulysine 206
    infusion of 207
    lispro 206
    mixtures 206
    resistance 208
    secretagogues 209
    sensitizers 209
    soluble 210
    therapy
        complications of 208
        methods of 207
    types 206
Insulin-dependent diabetes, contraindicated in 143
Intercostal muscles 126
Intestine 5
Intracranial pressure 40
Intragastric pressure, increased 60
Intraocular pressure, increased 60
Intravenous
    agents 221
    anesthesia, total 42
    anesthetic
        agents 35, 42*t*
        comparison of 36*t*
    bioavailability of 2
    bolus 188
Inverse agonists 8
Iodides 212
Ion-channel receptor 8, 13
Ionotropes 131

Ionotropic agents 150*t*
Ipratropium bromide 65, 117
Irbesartan 172
Iron 114
Ischemic heart disease 76, 143, 182
  drugs in 160
Isoflurane 30
Isoprenaline 120, 132
Itopride 108
Itraconazole 114

J

Junctional premature beat 181

K

Kent's bundle 184
Ketaconazole 17
Ketamine 39, 40, 42, 205
Ketoconazole 114
Ketoprofen 75
Ketorolac 74
Kidney 15, 22, 225
  action in 70

L

Labetalol 230
Labor, effects on 70
Lansoprazole 67, 110, 112
Laryngospasm, severe 230
Left bundle branch block 178
Lenegre's disease 179
Lepirudin 189
Leukopenia 112
Leukotriene antagonists 118
Leukotriene inhibitors, pathway of 124*fc*
Leukotriene pathway inhibitors 123
Leukotriene receptor antagonists 124
Levodopa 15, 195
  adverse effects of 196
Levorphanol 79
Lidocaine 4, 89, 91, 186
Lignocaine 88, 92
Limb paresthesia 95
Lipopolysaccharides 129
Lipoxygenase inhibitors 123
Lisinopril 151, 157, 170
Lithium 208
Liver 5, 220

damage, allergic 22
disease 17
  chronic 225
  severe 5
dysfunction 225
Local anesthetics 87, 91*t*
  comparison of characteristics of 92*t*
Loop diuretics 154, 162, 166
Lorazepam 49, 52, 102, 205, 226
Losartan 151
Lown-Ganong-Levine syndrome 184
Loxatidine 110
Lungs 5

M

Magnesium hydroxide 114
Malathion 61
Maprotiline 201
Marcaine 92
Mast cell stabilizers 123
Meclizine 105, 108
Medicine 1
Meglitinides 208
Melatonin congener 47
Meperidine 82
Mephentermine 149, 150
Mepivacaine 88
Mesalamine 72
Metabolic acidemia 220
Metabolic acidosis 222
Metabolic effects 142
Metabolism
  bypass first-pass 6
  first-pass 5
  sites of first-pass 5
Metaprolol 17, 156
Metaraminol 149
Metformin 209
Methadone 79, 83
Methohexital 205
Methoxyflurane 17
Methylated xanthine alkaloids 120
Methylation 18
Methyldopa 151, 226
Methyl-morphine 82
Methylsalicylate 72
Methylxanthines 120
Metoclopramide 102, 108, 232
Metocurine 53, 55

Metolazone 163
Metoprolol 144
Metronidazole 17
Mexiletine 186
Mianserin 200
Midazolam 41, 42, 44, 52, 67
Midodrine 149
Migraine prophylaxis 143
Milk alkali syndrome 114
Milrinone 131, 132, 149
Minoxidil 137, 151, 157
Mirtazapine 200
Mitral valvular disease 182
Mivacurium 53, 55
Molecular weight heparin, low 188, 189
Monoamine oxidase inhibitors 67, 201, 203
Monooxygenases 16
Montelukast 124
   sodium 117
Moricizine 186
Morphine 78, 79, 81
   uses of 84
Mosapride 106, 108
Motilides 106
Moxonidine 151, 159
Mucokinetics 127
Mucolytics 126, 127
Muscarinic cholinergic receptors 9
Muscarinic receptor 8
   antagonists 198
Muscle
   relaxants 53, 55t
      depolarizing 53
   smooth 12
   type receptor 14
Mutagenesis 21
Myalgia 60
Myasthenia gravis 63
Myocardial infarction 143
   acute 129, 138, 160, 230
Myocardial ischemia, pathophysiology of 161f
Myocardial myofilament 219
Myoglobinuria 60

N

Nadolol 156
Nalbuphine 85
Nalmephine 86
Nalorphine 86
Naloxone 81, 85
Naltrexone 81, 85
Naproxen 75
Nateglinide 209
Nausea 25, 95, 101
   drugs in 101
Nebivolol 144
Nebulizers 216, 217
Nedocromil sodium 123
Neostigmine 61, 63
Nephrotic syndrome 163
Nephrotoxicity 21
Nerve
   growth factor receptor 8
   stimulators 58
Neurodegenerative disorders 217
Neuromuscular block monitoring 57
Neuromuscular blockade 58
Neuromuscular monitoring 57f
New York Heart Association 144
Nicardipine 158, 174, 230
Nicotamide adenine dinucleotide phosphate 16
Nicotinic acetylcholine receptor 14f
Nicotinic cholinergic receptors 13
Nicotinic receptor 13
Nifedipine 134, 158, 174, 208
Nimodipine 174
Nitrates 160
Nitrazepam 49, 52, 228
Nitric oxide 34, 129
Nitroglycerin 230
Nitroprusside 151, 157
Nitrous oxide 32, 44
Nonbenzodiazepines 47
Noncovalent reactions 21
Nondepolarizing block, characteristics of 56
Nondepolarizing muscle 54
   relaxants 53
Non-dihydropyridines 174
Nondrug regimen 152
Nonhemolytic jaundice, congenital 17
Nonopioids 128
Nonparoxysmal junctional tachycardia 182

Nonreceptor-mediated drug action 13
Nonsteroidal anti-inflammatory drugs
   adverse effects of 77
   pharmacokinetics of 70
Noradrenaline 131, 132, 147, 150
Norepinephrine reuptake inhibitors 200
Nortriphyline 201
Nuclear receptor 8

O

Obstructive lung disease, chronic 81
Obstructive pulmonary disease, chronic 66
Olsalazine 72
Omalizumab 124
Omeprazole 17
Ondansetron 67, 103, 108
Onium chlorofumarate, mixed 53
Opiates 128
Opioid 233
   antagonists 85
   centrally acting 78
   clinical uses of 86
   comparison of 81*t*
   receptor 79
      agonists, comparison of 79*t*
Oral anticoagulants, newer 191
Oral antidiabetic agents 208
   classification 208
Oral glucocorticoids 122
Osmotic diuretics 164
Oxaprozin 75
Oxazepam 226
Oxeladin 128
Oxicams 69, 75
Oxide 52
Oxygen 34
   delivery systems 214
   head hood 214
   incubator 214
   therapy
      advantages of 213
      and humidification 213
      clinical guidance for 214
      evaluation of effectiveness of 214
      hazards of 214
      long-term 214
      techniques of 213

P

Pain, prevention of 59
Palonosetron 104
Pancuronium 55
Pantoprazole 67, 110, 112
Paracetamol 17, 72, 226
Paraldehyde 46
Parenteral anesthetics 35
Parenteral anticoagulants 189
Parenteral glucocorticoids 122
Parkinson's disease 197
Parkinsonism, drugs in 195
Parnaparin 189
Paroxetine 200
Pentazocine 67, 81, 84
Peptic ulcer disease 109
   classification 109
   drugs in 109
Perindopril 170
Peripheral anticholinergic action 198
Peripheral nerves 12
Peripheral resistance, total 135
Pethidine 67, 81, 82
Pharmacodynamics, age-related changes in 227
Pharmacokinetics 54
   age-related changes in 227
Pharyngeal demulcents 126, 127
Phenobarbitone 17, 51
Phenothiazines 114
Phentolamine 230
Phenylbutazone 17
Phenylephrine 148
Phenytoin
   causes 205
   decreases manifestations 17
Phenytoxin 17
Pheochromocytoma 143
Phosphodiesterase inhibitors 132, 166
Physostigmine 1, 61, 63, 232
Pioglitazone 209
Piperazines, tricyclic 199
Plasma 15
   cholinesterase antagonism 59
   protein 220
   replacement fluid 130
Platelet
   action on 70
   inhibitors 191

Poisoning, chronic 17
Postspinal headache 98, 99
   mechanism of 99
Postsuccinylcholine muscle pain 59
Potassium-sparing diuretics 154, 162, 163
Pramlintide 209
Pranlukast 124
Prasugrel 192
Prazosin 151, 156
Preanesthetic medications 67
Precordial discomfort 95
Preexcitation syndrome 183
Pregnidoxin 108
Prinzmetal's angina 143
Procainamide 186
Procaine 15, 88, 90, 91, 93
Prodrugs 16
Prokinetic agents 101, 105
Prolactin receptor 8
Proopiomelanocortin 78
Propafenone 186
Propanolol 156
Propidium 61
Propionic acid derivatives 69, 75
Propofol 37, 40, 42, 44, 205
Propranalol 4, 5, 144, 186, 230
Propylthiouracil 232
Prostaglandin 69
   analogs 112
Protamine sulfate 191, 232
Protein 219
Proton pump inhibitors 67, 111
Prototype drug atropine, actions of 65
Protriptyline 201
Prucalopride 106
Pruritus 222
Pulmonary absorption collapse 215
Pulmonary edema 231
   management 231
Pulmonary hypertension, drugs in 161
Pulmonary system 225
Pulmonary toxicity 215
Pump failure, treatment of 160
Pyrazolone derivatives 69
Pyridostigmine 61, 63
Pyrrolopyrole 69

Q

Quinidine 17, 186
Quinine 1

R

Rabeprazole 110, 112
Ramipril 157, 170
Ranitidine 67, 110
Rash 172
Reactions
   covalent 21
   type A 20
   type B 20
Regional anesthesia 94, 96
   advantages 94
   characteristics of 94t
   disadvantages 95
Remifentanil 83
Renal disease 5
Renal failure, chronic 222
Renal function 219
   altered 168
   dose calculation in impaired 224
Renin inhibitor, direct 153
Renin-angiotensin system
   components of 166
   effects of 168
   functions of 168
   mechanism of action of 168fc
   pathophysiology of 166
Repaglinide 209
Respiratory changes 222
Respiratory components in neonate and adult 218t
Respiratory rate 40
Respiratory system 24, 49, 146, 218
Respiratory tract 66, 142
Restlessness 95
Reteplase 193
Retrolental fibroplasia 215
Reviparin 189
Reye's syndrome 71, 72
Rheumatic disease 72
Rifampicin 17
Right bundle branch block 178
Rivaroxaban 191
Rocuronium 55
Ropivacaine 91, 93
Roxatidine 110
Ryanodine 144

S

Salbutamol 117, 208
Salicylates 69, 226

Salicylic acid 72
Salmeterol 120
Saxagliptin 209
Scopolamine 184
Second messenger 18
Sedative 46
Sensitive potassium channels 13
Sensorcaine 92
Septic shock, treatment of 133
Serotonin
    reuptake inhibitors, selective 200, 201
    selective 200
    transporter 201
Sertraline 200
Serum cholinesterase, low 59
Sevoflurane 32
Shock 129
    anaphylactic 22, 129
    cardiogenic 129, 132
    compensatory mechanisms 130
    hypovolemic 129
    mechanisms responsible for 129
    neurogenic 130
    pathophysiology of 129
    septic 129
    treatment of 129, 130
    types of 129
Sick sinus syndrome 175, 181, 182
Sincalide 107
Sinus
    bradycardia 180
    tachycardia 180
Sitagliptin 209
Skeletal muscle 54
    relaxants 53
Skin 5
Smooth muscles, action on 66
Sodium
    bicarbonate 114
    cromoglycate 117
    nitroprusside 134, 230
Sotalol 186
Spinal analgesia, drugs for 98
Spinal anesthesia
    cephalad migration of 130
    complications of 95t
    prevention of hypotension to 96
    total 100
    treatment of hypotension to 96

Spinal block
    analgesia in 98
    high 95
Spinal over epidural anesthesia, disadvantages of 96
Spironolactone 163
Stable angina 160
Status asthmaticus, treatment of 125
Steroid 226
    hormones 8
    withdrawal, signs of 123
Streptokinase 193
Strophanthin G 176
Subarachnoid block, contraindications for 96
Succinylcholine 15, 54, 55
    adverse effects of 60
    apnea 58
Sucralfate 113
Sufentanil 79
Sugamadex 63
Sulfated glycosaminoglycan 187
Sulfonal 46
Sulfonylureas 208
Sulindac 73
Supraventricular tachycardia, paroxysmal 175, 181
Sweat glands and temperature, action on 66
Sympathomimetic
    characteristics of 131t
    drugs 180, 203
Systemic embolization, danger of 182
Systemic lupus erythematosus, drug-induced 22
Systemic steroids, side effects of 123
Systemic vascular resistance 225
Systolic blood pressure 147

T

Tachycardia 120
Tacrine 17, 61
Telmisartan 151, 172
Temazepam 52
Temperature regulation 220
Tenecteplase 193
Teratogenesis 21
Terazosin 151, 156

Testosterone 15
Tetracaine 91
Tetracyclines 114, 226
Thebaine 78
Theophylline 17, 208
Therapeutic gases 34
Thevetia 176
Thiazides 154, 162, 163, 208
Thiazolidinediones 208
Thienopyridine 192
Thioamides 211
Thiopentone 40, 51
Thoracic surgery 182
Thyroid
   disorder 212
      drugs in 211
   storm 232
Thyrotoxicosis 143
Tianeptine 200
Ticlopidine 192
Tiotropium bromide 65
Tocainide 186
Tolbutamide 17
Tolmetin 74
Torsades de pointes, treatment of 132
Torsemide 163
Toxicity 215
Tramadol 67, 81, 83
Transmembrane enzyme 8
Transtracheal oxygen delivery 214
Trazodone 200
Triamterene 163
Trihexyphenidyl 198
Trimethaphan 230
Tubocurarine 55

U

Urethane 46
Urinary bladder, action on 66

Urokinase 193
Urticaria 111

V

Valsartan 172
Vasopressin antagonists 165
Vasopressor therapy 232
Vecuronium 14, 53, 55, 56, 63, 205
Ventricular failure, left 136
Ventricular fibrillation 183
Ventricular premature beats 182
   appearance of 183
Ventricular tachycardia 183
Verapamil 158, 174, 175, 186
Vildagliptin 209
Vitamin
   D 8, 15
   K antagonists 190
Vomiting 25, 95, 101
   drugs in 101
   mechanism of 102f

W

Warfarin 17, 190, 233
Wolff-Parkinson-White syndrome 177, 181, 183, 185, 186

X

Xenon 33

Z

Zafirlukast 124
Zaleplon 47
Z-compounds 47
Zileuton 123
Zolpidem 47, 52
Zopiclone 47, 51

EU GSPR Authorised Reprsentative
Logos Europe, 9 rue Nicolas Poussin
1700, La Rochelle, France
Phone: +33 (0) 6 67 93 73 78
E-mail: contact@logoseurope.eu